PRE-HOSPITAL PAEDIATRIC LIFE SUPPORT

PRE-HOSPITAL PAEDIATRIC LIFE SUPPORT

Advanced Life Support Group

First published in 1999
by BMJ Books, BMA House, Tavistock Square,
London WC1H 9JR

British Library Cataloguing in Publication Data

A catalogue record for this book is available from the British Library

ISBN 0-7279-1419-7

Typeset in Great Britain by Latimer Trend & Company Ltd, Plymouth
Printed and bound in Spain by GraphyCems

CONTENTS

CONTENTS

PART V: PRACTICAL PROCEDURES

PART VI: APPENDICES

WORKING GROUP

A sub-group of the
Advanced Paediatric Life Support (APLS)
Working Group

Tim Hodgetts	Accident & Emergency, Frimley Park
Fiona Jewkes	Paediatric Nephrology, Cardiff
Paul Lubas	Resuscitation Training/Paramedic, Cardiff
Kevin McCusker	Resuscitation Training/Paramedic, Cardiff
Peter Oakley	Anaesthetics/Trauma, Stoke
Joan Robson	Paediatric Accident & Emergency, Liverpool
Susan Wieteska	International Coordinator, Manchester

CONTRIBUTORS

Tim Hodgetts   Accident & Emergency, Frimley

Fiona Jewkes   Paediatric Nephrology, Cardiff

Sarah Levene   Child Accident Prevention Trust, London

Paul Lubas   Resuscitation Training/Ex-paramedic, Cardiff

Kevin McCusker Resuscitation Training/Ex-paramedic, Cardiff

Peter Oakley   Anaesthetics/Trauma, Stoke

Joan Robson   Paediatric Accident & Emergency, Liverpool

PREFACE

Pre-hospital Paediatric Life Support: The Practical Approach was written as a sister publication to *Advanced Paediatric Life Support: The Practical Approach*. It has the same objective of improving the emergency care of children, but concentrates on the first critical minutes prior to arriving at hospital.

It has been developed to fill a void in the training of personnel who have sometimes had to deal with these children with little knowledge or experience of paediatrics. Members of the pre-hospital life support working group, all of whom have extensive experience of working with children in both the pre-hospital and the hospital environments, have developed the manual in conjunction with the Joint Colleges and Ambulance Liaison Committee (JCALC) working party on paediatrics.

This manual also forms the core text of the PHPLS course, which is designed to give both medical and paramedical staff the skills and knowledge to deal with paediatric trauma and medical emergencies. The editors feel that by training together these multidisciplinary groups will both complement each other and reduce potential barriers thus developing a seamless care approach to these events.

The course is designed to dovetail with the therapies presented in APLS, building upon established and tested interventions that we hope will ultimately provide an improvement in patient outcomes.

The layout of this book begins with background information on the aetiology of illness and disease in children, followed by the assessment and basic life support of children. Specific pre-hospital considerations are then covered followed by practical skills to apply your new-found knowledge.

Emergencies in children can generate a great deal of anxiety in the children, parents and medical personnel who have to deal with them. We hope that this book will enlighten the reader on the subject of pre-hospital paediatric emergency care and provide some support to help all involved. Read it as part of the PHPLS course or as a stand-alone publication, refer to it frequently, and hopefully it will help to achieve its aim of improving the standards of paediatric life support within the pre-hospital setting.

Fiona Jewkes
Paul Lubas
Kevin McCusker
(*Editorial Board*)

December 1998

ACKNOWLEDGEMENTS

A great many people have put a lot of hard work into the production of this book, and the accompanying pre-hospital paediatric life support course. The editors would like to thank all the contributors for their efforts together with the contributors to the *Advanced Paediatric Life Support: The Practical Approach* text and course to which the Pre-hospital text and course is closely aligned. We would also like to thank all the PHPLS instructors and candidates who took the time to send their comments to us.

We are greatly indebted to Helen Carruthers and Mary Harrison MMAA for producing the excellent line drawings that illustrate the text. Thanks also to the Welsh Ambulance Service for their help with the cover and to Ian Maconochie for his help with the proof reading.

Finally, we would like to thank, in advance, those of you who will attend the Pre-hospital Paediatric Life Support course in the future; no doubt, you will have much constructive criticism to offer.

PART

I

INTRODUCTION

CHAPTER

1

Introduction

CAUSES OF DEATH IN CHILDHOOD

As can be seen from Table 1.1, the greatest mortality during childhood occurs in the first year of life, with the highest death rate of all happening in the first month.

Table 1.1. Number of deaths by age group

Age group	Number of deaths
0–28 days	2534
1–52 weeks	1291
1–4 years	720
5–14 years	984

England and Wales, 1997: Office for National Statistics

The causes of death vary with age, as shown in Table 1.2. In the newborn period the commonest causes are congenital abnormalities and factors associated with prematurity such as respiratory immaturity, cerebral haemorrhage, and infection due to immaturity of the immune response.

From one month to one year of age the condition called "cot death" is the most common cause of death. Some victims of this condition have previously unrecognised respiratory or metabolic disease, but some have no specific cause of death found at detailed post-mortem examination. This latter group is described as suffering from the Sudden Infant Death syndrome. There has been a striking reduction in the incidence of cot death over the past few years in the UK, Holland, Australia, and New Zealand.

Table 1.2. Common causes of death by age group

Cause	Number (%) of deaths at		
	4–52 weeks	1–4 years	5–14 years
Cot death	324 (25)	4 (1)	0 (0)
Congenital abnormality	253 (18)	123 (17)	72 (7)
Infection	126 (10)	59 (8)	85 (9)
Trauma	64 (5)	114 (16)	292[a] (30)
Neoplasms	26 (2)	93 (13)	224 (23)

England and Wales, 1997: Office for National Statistics
[a] Includes 2 suicides/self-inflicted injury.

3

In England and Wales the decrease has been from 1597 in 1988, 454 in 1994 to 328 in 1997. The reduction has followed national campaigns to inform parents of known risk factors such as the prone sleeping position in the infant and parental smoking. The next most common causes of death in this age group are congenital abnormalities and infections.

Between the ages of 1 and 4 years, congenital abnormality and trauma are about equally split and after 4 years of age trauma is the most frequent cause of death, and remains so until well into adult life. Deaths from trauma have been described as falling into three groups. The first group suffer overwhelming damage at the time of the trauma and the injury caused is incompatible with life; children with these massive injuries will die within minutes, whatever is done. The second group die because of progressive respiratory failure, circulatory insufficiency or raised intracranial pressure secondary to the effects of injury; death occurs within a few hours if no treatment is administered, but can be avoided if treatment is prompt and effective. The final group consists of late deaths due to raised intracranial pressure, infection or multiple organ failure. Appropriate management in the first few hours will decrease mortality in this group also. The trimodal distribution of trauma deaths is illustrated in Figure 1.1.

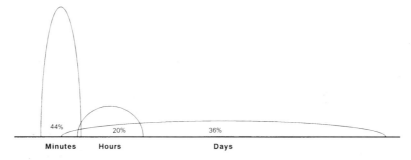

Figure 1.1.   Trimodal distribution of trauma deaths

Only a minority of deaths in childhood, such as those due to unresponsive end stage neoplastic disease, are expected and "managed". Most children with potentially fatal diseases such as complex congenital heart disease, inborn errors of metabolism or cystic fibrosis are treated or "cured" by operation, diet, transplant or, soon, even gene therapy. The approach to these children is to treat vigorously incidental illnesses (such as respiratory infections) to which many are especially prone. Therefore, some children who present to hospital with serious life threatening acute illness also have an underlying chronic disease.

PATHWAYS LEADING TO CARDIORESPIRATORY ARREST

Cardiac arrest in infancy and childhood is rarely due to primary cardiac disease. This is different from the situation in adults where the primary arrest is often cardiac, and cardiorespiratory function may remain near normal until the moment that the arrest occurs. In childhood most cardiac arrests are secondary to hypoxia. Underlying causes include birth asphyxia, epiglottitis, inhalation of foreign body, bronchiolitis, asthma and pneumothorax. Respiratory arrest also occurs secondarily to neurological dysfunction such as that caused by some poisons or during convulsions. Raised intracranial pressure due to head injury or acute encephalopathy eventually leads to respiratory arrest, but severe neuronal damage has already been sustained before the arrest occurs.

Whatever the cause, by the time cardiac arrest occurs the child has had a period of respiratory insufficiency which will have caused hypoxia and respiratory and metabolic acidosis. The combination of hypoxia and acidosis causes cell damage and death (particularly in more sensitive organs such as the brain, liver, and kidney) before myocardial damage is severe enough to cause cardiac arrest.

Most other cardiac arrests are secondary to circulatory failure (shock). This will have resulted either from fluid or blood loss or from fluid maldistribution within the circulatory system. The former may be due to gastroenteritis, burns or trauma while the latter is often caused by sepsis, heart failure or anaphylaxis. As all organs are deprived of essential nutrients and oxygen as shock progresses to cardiac arrest, circulatory failure like respiratory failure, causes tissue hypoxia and acidosis. In fact, both pathways may occur in the same condition. The pathways leading to cardiac arrest in children are summarised in Figure 1.2.

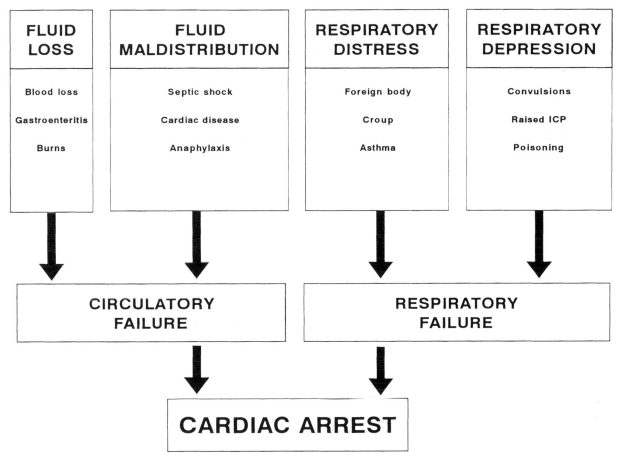

Figure 1.2. Pathways to cardiac arrest in childhood (with examples of underlying causes)

The worst outcome is in children who have had an out-of-hospital arrest and who arrive apnoeic and pulseless. These children have a poor chance of intact neurological survival. There has often been a prolonged period of hypoxia and ischaemia before the start of adequate cardiopulmonary resuscitation (CPR). Earlier recognition of seriously ill children and paediatric cardiopulmonary resuscitation training for the public could improve the outcome for these children.

2

Why treat children differently?

OBJECTIVES

After reading this chapter you should be able to:

- Calculate a child's weight from their age
- Identify the differences in anatomy and physiology of airway, breathing, and circulation at different ages
- Discuss the psychological differences between adults and children

INTRODUCTION

Children are not little adults. The spectrum of diseases that they suffer from is different, and their responses to disease and injury may differ both physically and psychologically. This chapter deals with some specific points that have particular relevance to emergency care.

SIZE

The most obvious reason for treating children differently is their size, and its variation with age.

Weight

The most rapid changes in size occur in the first year of life. An average birth weight of 3.5 kg has increased to 10.3 kg by the age of 1 year. After that time weight increases more slowly until the pubertal growth spurt. This is illustrated in the weight chart for boys shown in Figure 2.1.

As most therapies are given as a dose per kilogram, it is important to get some idea of a child's weight as soon as possible. In the emergency situation this is especially difficult because it is often impracticable to weigh the child. To overcome this problem a number of methods can be used to derive a weight estimate.

If the age is known the formula:

$$\text{Weight (kg)} = 2 \, (\text{age in years} + 4)$$

can be used if the child is aged between 1 and 10 years old. If the child is less than 1 year, he or she will double their birth weight by 6 months and treble it by 1 year. In

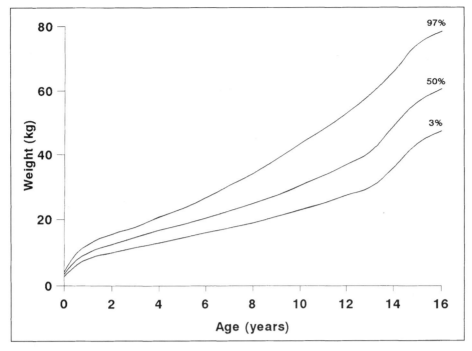

Figure 2.1. Weight chart for boys

addition, various charts (such as the Oakley chart) (Figure 2.2) are available which allow an approximation of weight to be derived from the age. Finally the Broselow tape (which relates weight to height) can be used. Whatever the method, it is essential that the carer is sufficiently familiar with it to be able to use it quickly and accurately.

Body proportions

The body proportions change with age. This is most graphically illustrated by considering the body surface area (BSA). At birth the head accounts for 19% of BSA; this falls to 9% by the age of 15 years. Figure 2.3 shows these changes.

The BSA to weight ratio decreases with age. Small children, with a high ratio, lose heat more rapidly and consequently are relatively more prone to hypothermia.

Certain specific changes in body proportions also have a bearing on emergency care. For example, the relatively large head and short neck of the infant tend to cause neck flexion and this, together with the relatively large tongue, make airway care difficult. Specific problems such as this are highlighted in the relevant chapters.

ANATOMY AND PHYSIOLOGY

Particular anatomical and physiological features, and the way they change with age, can have a bearing on emergency care. Although there are changes in most areas, the most important from this perspective are those that occur in the respiratory and cardiovascular systems. These are discussed in more detail below.

Anatomy

Airway

Anatomical features outside the airway have some relevance to its care. As mentioned above the head is large and the neck short, tending to cause neck flexion. The face and mandible are small and teeth or orthodontic appliances may be loose. The relatively large tongue not only tends to obstruct the airway in an unconscious child, but may

Paediatric resuscitation chart

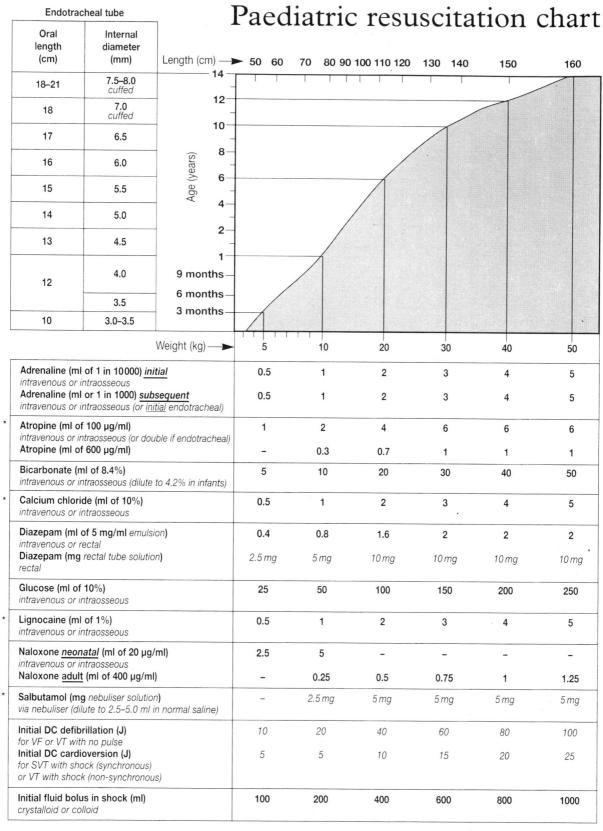

Endotracheal tube

Oral length (cm)	Internal diameter (mm)
18–21	7.5–8.0 cuffed
18	7.0 cuffed
17	6.5
16	6.0
15	5.5
14	5.0
13	4.5
12	4.0
	3.5
10	3.0–3.5

Weight (kg) ➤	5	10	20	30	40	50
Adrenaline (ml of 1 in 10000) *initial* intravenous or intraosseous	0.5	1	2	3	4	5
Adrenaline (ml or 1 in 1000) *subsequent* intravenous or intraosseous (or *initial* endotracheal)	0.5	1	2	3	4	5
* **Atropine (ml of 100 µg/ml)** intravenous or intraosseous (or double if endotracheal)	1	2	4	6	6	6
Atropine (ml of 600 µg/ml)	–	0.3	0.7	1	1	1
Bicarbonate (ml of 8.4%) intravenous or intraosseous (dilute to 4.2% in infants)	5	10	20	30	40	50
* **Calcium chloride (ml of 10%)** intravenous or intraosseous	0.5	1	2	3	4	5
Diazepam (ml of 5 mg/ml *emulsion***)** intravenous or rectal	0.4	0.8	1.6	2	2	2
Diazepam (mg *rectal tube solution***)** rectal	2.5 mg	5 mg	10 mg	10 mg	10 mg	10 mg
Glucose (ml of 10%) intravenous or intraosseous	25	50	100	150	200	250
* **Lignocaine (ml of 1%)** intravenous or intraosseous	0.5	1	2	3	4	5
Naloxone *neonatal* **(ml of 20 µg/ml)** intravenous or intraosseous	2.5	5	–	–	–	–
Naloxone *adult* **(ml of 400 µg/ml)**	–	0.25	0.5	0.75	1	1.25
* **Salbutamol (mg** *nebuliser solution***)** via nebuliser (dilute to 2.5–5.0 ml in normal saline)	–	2.5 mg	5 mg	5 mg	5 mg	5 mg
Initial DC defibrillation (J) for VF or VT with no pulse	10	20	40	60	80	100
Initial DC cardioversion (J) for SVT with shock (synchronous) or VT with shock (non-synchronous)	5	5	10	15	20	25
Initial fluid bolus in shock (ml) crystalloid or colloid	100	200	400	600	800	1000

* **CAUTION!**   *Non-standard drug concentrations may be available:*
*Use **Atropine** 100 µg/ml or prepare by diluting 1 mg to 10 ml or 600 µg to 6 ml in normal saline.*
*Note that 1 ml of **calcium chloride** 10% is equivalent to 3 ml of **calcium gluconate** 10%.*
*Use **Lignocaine** (without adrenaline) 1% or give twice the volume of 0.5%. Give half the volume of 2% or dilute appropriately.*
***Salbutamol** may also be given by slow intravenous injection (4–6 µg/kg), but beware of the different concentrations available (eg 50 and 500 µg/ml).*

Figure 2.2.   Oakley chart

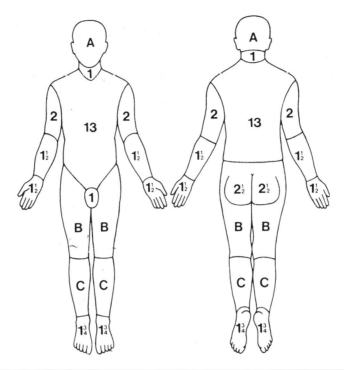

	Surface area at				
Area indicated	0	1 year	5 years	10 years	15 years
A	9.5	8.5	6.5	5.5	4.5
B	2.75	3.25	4.0	4.5	4.5
C	2.5	2.5	2.75	3.0	3.25

Figure 2.3. Body surface area (%). (Reproduced courtesy of Smith & Nephew Pharmaceutical Ltd)

also impede the view at laryngoscopy. Finally the floor of the mouth is easily compressible, requiring care in the positioning of fingers when holding the jaw for airway positioning. These features are summarised in Figure 2.4.

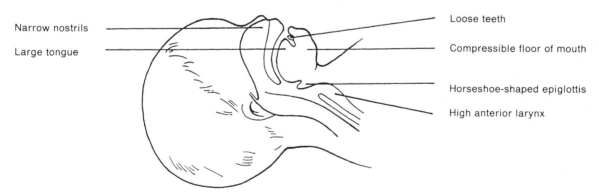

Figure 2.4. Summary of significant upper airway anatomy

The anatomy of the airway itself changes with age, and consequently different problems affect different age groups. Infants less than 6 months old are obligate nasal breathers. As the narrow nasal passages are easily obstructed by mucous secretions, and upper respiratory tract infections are common in this age group, these children are at particular risk of airway compromise. In 3- to 8-year-olds adenotonsillar hypertrophy is a problem. This not only tends to cause obstruction, but also causes difficulty when the nasal route is used to pass pharyngeal, gastric or tracheal tubes.

9

In all young children the epiglottis is horseshoe-shaped, and projects posteriorly at 45° making tracheal intubation more difficult. This, together with the fact that the larynx is high and anterior (at the level of the second and third cervical vertebrae in the infant, compared with the fifth and sixth vertebrae in the adult), means that it is easier to intubate an infant using a straight-bladed laryngoscope. The cricoid ring is the narrowest part of the upper airway (as opposed to the larynx in an adult) and the surrounding tissues are particularly susceptible to oedema. Since endotracheal tube cuffs tend to lie at this level, uncuffed tubes are preferred in pre-pubertal children.

The trachea is short and soft. Over-extension of the neck therefore may cause tracheal compression. The short trachea and the symmetry of the carinal angles mean that not only is tube displacement more likely, but also a tube or a foreign body is just as likely to be displaced into the left as the right main stem bronchus.

Breathing

The lungs are relatively immature at birth, and increase in the number of small airways from birth to adulthood. Both the upper and lower airways are relatively small. They are consequently more easily obstructed. Seemingly small obstructions can have significant effects on air entry in children.

Infants rely mainly on diaphragmatic breathing and their muscles are more likely to fatigue compared with adults. Pre-term infants' muscles tire even more easily. These children are consequently more prone to respiratory failure.

The ribs lie more horizontally in infants, and therefore contribute less to chest expansion. In the injured child, the compliant chest wall may allow serious underlying lung injuries to occur without necessarily incurring rib fractures. For multiple rib fractures to occur the force must be very large; the parenchymal injury that results is consequently very severe and flail chest is tolerated badly.

Circulation

At birth the two cardiac ventricles are of similar weight; by 2 months of age the left ventricle is significantly heavier than the right. These changes are reflected in the infant's ECG. During the first months of life the right ventricle (RV) dominance is apparent, but by 4–6 months of age the left ventricle (LV) is dominant. As the heart develops during childhood the size of the P wave and QRS complex increase, and the P–R interval and QRS duration become longer.

The child's circulating blood volume is higher per kilogram body weight (70–80 ml/kg) than that of an adult, but the actual volume is small. This means that in infants and small children relatively small absolute amounts of blood loss can be critically important.

Physiology

Airway and Breathing

The infant has a relatively greater metabolic rate and oxygen consumption. This is one reason for an increased respiratory rate (see Table 2.1). However, the tidal volume remains relatively constant in relation to body weight (5–7 ml/kg) through to adulthood.

Table 2.1. Respiratory rate by age

Age (years)	Respiratory rate (breaths per minute)
<1	30–40
2–5	25–30
5–12	20–25
>12	15–20

The child's compliant chest wall leads to prominent sternal recession and rib space indrawing when the airway is obstructed or lung compliance decreases. It also allows the intrathoracic pressure to be less "negative". This reduces small airway patency. As a result, the lung volume at end expiration is similar to the closing volume (the volume at which small airway closure starts to take place).

Circulation

The heart rate decreases with age, as shown in Table 2.2.

Table 2.2. Heart rate by age

Age (years)	Heart rate (beats per minute)
<1	110–160
2–5	95–140
5–12	80–120
>12	60–100

The amount of blood pumped with each contraction of the ventricles (the stroke volume) is relatively fixed in infants compared to older children and adults. Thus if fluid is put into the circulation, an older child is able to increase the amount of blood pumped with each contraction, in addition to the circulation being increased by the extra volume. However, the response in a baby is limited to that of volume expansion. This means that if fluid is given to resuscitate a baby, they will not respond as well as an adult or older child. By the age of 2 years the cardiac function is similar to an adult.

Systemic vascular resistance rises after birth and continues to do so until adulthood is reached. This is reflected in the changes seen in blood pressure, shown in Table 2.3.

Table 2.3. Systolic blood pressure by age

Age (years)	Systolic blood pressure (mmHg)
<1	70–90
2–5	80–100
5–12	90–110
>12	100–120

PSYCHOLOGY

Children who are ill or injured present particular problems during emergency management because of the difficulties in communication with them, and because of the fear that they feel.

Communication

Infants and young children have either no language ability, or are still developing their speech. This causes difficulty when symptoms such as pain need to be described. Even children who are usually fluent may remain silent. Information has to be gleaned from the limited verbal communication, and from the many non-verbal cues (such as facial expression and posture) that are available.

Fear

All emergency situations, and many other situations that adults would not classify as emergencies, produce fear in children. This causes additional distress to the child and adds to parental anxiety. Physiological parameters, such as pulse rate and respiratory rate, are altered because of it, and this in turn makes clinical assessment more difficult.

Fear is a particular problem in the pre-school child who often has a "magical" concept of illness and injury. This means that the child often feels that the problem has been caused by some bad wish or thought that they have had. School age children and adolescents may have fearsome concepts of what might happen to them because of ideas they have picked up from adult conversation, films, and television.

Knowledge allays fear and it is therefore important to explain things as clearly as possible to the child. Explanations must be phrased in a way that the child can understand. Play can be used to do this (eg applying a bandage to a teddy first), and also helps to maintain some semblance of normality in a strange and stressful situation. Finally parents must be allowed to stay with the child at all times; their absence from the bedside will only add additional fears both to the child and to the parents themselves. Involving the parents in simple tasks will also be helpful as many will feel very helpless in a time of medical emergency for the child.

SUMMARY

- Absolute size and relative body proportions change with age.
- Charts and formulae are available to assist in the estimation of the child's weight.
- Observations on children must be related to their age.
- Therapy in children must be related to their age and weight.
- The special psychological needs of children must be considered.

Questions

1 Calculate the weight of an 8-year-old child, using an appropriate formula.
2 Why are uncuffed endotracheal tubes used in pre-pubertal children?
3 How can parents help a child psychologically in a medical emergency?

CHAPTER
3
Examining sick children

OBJECTIVES

After reading this chapter you should know how to approach and examine a:

- Baby
- Toddler
- School child/adolescent

ASSESSMENT

The general appearance of the child can give a rapid and surprisingly accurate assessment as to what kind of medical intervention is going to be required. A previously well 6-month-old baby who is lying floppy in his or her mother's arms, pale in colour and not interested in their surroundings is more likely to need urgent medical intervention and transport than a similarly aged baby who is pink and well perfused and who laughs and reaches out for toys. **Often, more valuable information can be learnt by merely observing a child than by trying to perform more detailed examinations**, as shown below in Table 3.1. This is particularly so in toddlers, who can be very difficult to examine because of their innate fear of strangers.

Table 3.1. Observations which can be made without touching a child

Airway	Noisy breathing, eg stridor
	Weak or strong cry
	Abnormal cry
Breathing	Unusual position (eg tripod position)
	Use of accessory muscles
	Recession
	Nasal flaring
	Grunting
Interaction with environment	Alertness, conscious level
	Readiness to play
	Interest in environment
Activity	Movement of limbs
	Spontaneously or only on stimulation?
Posture	Abnormal posture, eg neck retraction, hypotonia
	Decerebrate or decorticate posturing
Skin	Bruising
	Cyanosis
	Pallor
	Skin rash, eg petechiae/purpura

FURTHER EVALUATION

This will be dependent on the child's age. The examiner should try to work at the same height as the child—bending over a child may be very threatening. Smiling may be very reassuring.

Infants

Much reliance should again be placed on observation in this age group. Some babies will be crying already when you approach them, but others may be upset by an attempted removal of their clothes or by a cold stethoscope. In these situations more information can often be gained about the severity of the condition and the physical signs by just looking, than by more detailed assessment. During the general assessment a respiratory rate should be recorded.

In infants over the age of 6 or 7 months it may be better to conduct the examination, where possible, with the child on the parent's knee. Although this makes examination of some parts, such as the abdomen, difficult, it is still easier to examine a cooperative child in this position than to try to examine a hysterical child who has been prised away from his or her mother.

Generally it is better to examine the parts of the anatomy which require relative quiet first, in case the infant later becomes upset by the examination. This still allows assessment and examination of the airway, breathing, and circulation in the conventional order of ABC. The airway has already been examined by general observation and listening to the breathing, as has the work of breathing. Auscultation of the chest is best done early and allows an assessment of the effectiveness of the breathing. Feeling of the pulse, which also requires relative quiet and is best done at the brachial artery, can be done next, followed by an assessment of capillary refill. None of these things usually requires much exposure of the child, which may add to the child's insecurity and be upsetting.

Much assessment of disability has also already been done by general observation, but feeling the infant's fontanelle or "soft spot" can be a helpful additional sign. It is normally soft. Tension of the fontanelle may indicate raised intracranial pressure. The fontanelle will also become tense when the infant is crying. A sunken fontanelle may indicate dehydration.

It is not always appropriate or necessary to examine every infant from top to toe, exposing every inch of the body. Indeed it may actually be harmful, delaying transport and allowing the child to become cold and frightened. In older children, who sometimes feel insecure without all their clothing on or in cold environments, as much clothing should be kept on the child at any one time as is possible. One piece of clothing should be replaced before removing another in these circumstances. The exception is when the child feels very hot, in which case minimal loose clothing is appropriate to facilitate cooling.

Toddlers

Toddlers present many of the difficulties of younger infants during examination, but there are two extra points to remember.

First, they tend to be increasingly wary of strangers, and secondly, some children of this age can be particularly wilful and determined not to be examined. Generally this is a sign that they are not seriously ill and should be quite reassuring to the examiner, although it may be inconvenient. Often a gentle approach, at eye level (Figure 3.1), explaining to the child in terms he or she can understand may be adequately reassuring to allow examination. It is particularly important to get the parent to help you to reassure and to hold the child.

Allowing a frightened child to play with instruments which will be used, such as a stethoscope, can often avert the terror the child may experience if it is suddenly thrust upon the chest. If the child does become frightened and uncooperative it is generally best to restrict the examination to that which is absolutely essential. It may even be necessary to restrict one's examination to only that of the general appearance, as described above. This is particularly important when upper airway obstruction is being considered, as in croup and epiglottitis. Agitation may lead to complete airway obstruction and respiratory arrest in these circumstances. It is very important that no attempt is made to examine the mouth or throat if the child has stridor.

If the child does become agitated, it will only make matters worse if the examiner becomes impatient. To continue with kind words and smiles may do much more to alleviate the situation than showing the impatience which the examiner may be feeling. Even if the child is beyond reason, calm and caring behaviour will reassure the parent and this will undoubtedly help indirectly to reassure the child.

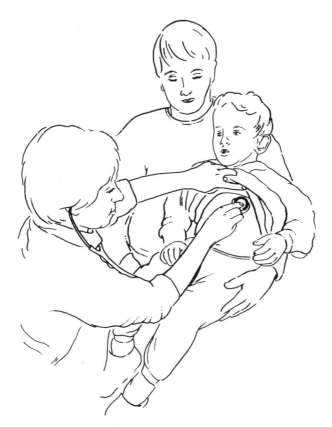

Figure 3.1. Examination of a small child

School children

As communication is easier in this group one would expect that cooperation would be greater, and in general it is. However, children sometimes regress in times of stress and become apparently quite unreasonable. In these circumstances it is important to remain patient and calm. If an older child seems unduly frightened he or she may be much happier sitting on a parent's knee and any apparent "babyish" behaviour should not be remarked upon. Remember that many of these children will have very mixed up emotions and fears linked to what has led to the accident or illness and they may be blaming themselves. Others will have had previous experience of the medical profession and may be frightened by uniforms or fearful of needles or pain because of past experience in health care settings.

Adolescents

One might imagine that adolescents would be as simple to examine as adults, but it must be remembered that they also have not reached either emotional or physical maturity. Whilst some may be mature and calm, others may be quite uncooperative. Often they are afraid to voice their anxieties, such as fear of death or losing a limb, in case they "look silly". It is important to remember to reassure this age group, despite their apparent maturity.

Some of these young people will have hidden agendas. It is possible that they should not have been where they were when the accident occurred, or perhaps their depressed conscious level is due to the ingestion of alcohol or drugs. Occasionally an adolescent will present with symptomatology which the examiner suspects is not due to a real physical problem, ie they are "putting it on". It is crucial to remember in these circumstances that the adolescent must be in quite some distress to have gone to these lengths and transportation to hospital and medical advice is clearly still appropriate. Confrontation and humiliation will not be helpful.

Finally, it is important to remember that young people in this group are often extremely shy of their developing bodies and every effort must be made to respect their wishes and preserve their modesty.

GENERAL IMPORTANT POINTS TO REMEMBER

1   Never lie to children. If you are going to hurt a child explain in an age-appropriate way the reason for needing to hurt and tell the child that the procedure will hurt. The first person that lies to a child about what is going to happen will lead to that child losing trust in all those subsequently caring for them. Lying should be avoided at all costs.

2   Always involve the parents. In the majority of age groups, having the child sit on a parent's knee or getting a parent to distract the child will not only help to reassure the child, but will make the parents feel that they are doing something, and this in itself will reassure both them and their child. (Remember parents often feel very helpless.)

3   Always try to keep the parents and the child together. A young child will not understand why his or her parents are being removed and the fears they already have will be compounded by the fact that they may fear they will never see their family again.

4   Never be angry with the child, however uncooperative he or she may become, while you are attempting to help them. Anger will not help to gain the child's cooperation, may distress them further and will almost certainly also distress the parents. Calm encouragement and a kindly smiling face will do a lot to reassure both the parents and the patient, however you are feeling.

5   Where possible, particularly in older children, always involve them in the discussions regarding their care if they are present in the room. Also remember that disabled children may comprehend more than you appreciate. It is very demeaning for a child to be totally ignored whilst the parents have the procedure explained to them. This attitude does not engender trust.

> **SUMMARY**
> - Much information can be gained from the general appearance of a child.
> - Always try to work at the child's eye level (if practical).
> - Evaluation of a child will differ depending on the child's age.

Questions

1 Describe four physical signs to assess breathing which can be observed without touching the child.
2 Name three abnormalities of posture which may be noted when examining a sick child.
3 What additional problems do toddlers present during examination compared to babies?

4

Scene management

OBJECTIVES

After reading this chapter you should know how to:

- Prioritise your actions at an incident involving children
- Assess the scene
- Communicate adequately with the hospital and other services
- Assess the need for triage

INTRODUCTION

Advanced life support training courses teach a systematic approach to the ill or injured patient following ABC guidelines. But the answer to the question, "What is your first priority at the scene?" is not "Airway", particularly when working in the pre-hospital arena. The first priority is to manage the scene, and then to manage individual casualties. A logical approach to scene management is essential in paediatric incidents, as it is very easy for emotions to cloud judgement when children are involved. This may endanger the rescuer, patient, and others alike.

A SYSTEMATIC APPROACH

A simple, systematic approach to the management of any incident can be remembered as **CONTROL then ACT**.

CONTROL the incident then

Assess
Communicate
Triage.

CONTROL of an incident is often implicit. When an ambulance is called to a child with an asthma attack at school there is the unspoken understanding of the teacher that the paramedic is in control of the situation. In some instances it may be necessary to assert authority and gain control of a group of people before being able to manage a casualty effectively—for example, a group of drunken youths outside a pub with a friend who has been assaulted.

Assessment includes the following:

- Safety—yourself, the scene, the casualties.
- Quick history.
- Reading the wreckage/scene.

Safety is paramount. Personal safety is assured by wearing appropriate protective clothing. For the ambulance service attending a child at home this may be no more than disposable latex gloves. At the scene of a road accident it may extend to a helmet (with integral visor, or separate safety glasses), and high-visibility durable clothing (usually including a motorway specification jacket, with either separate over-trousers or overalls). There are few ambulance services in the United Kingdom that offer suitable training or equipment for their staff to function in a chemical or fire environment.

Safety of the scene is achieved by parking to protect the scene. Where necessary, the police will be involved to safeguard personnel on the scene through traffic control and cordons, and will protect the forensic scene of crime.

Safety of any casualties should be subordinate to personal safety and scene safety. However, it is easy to imagine the situation where the temptation exists to rush in and help a vulnerable child at the expense of personal safety.

A quick history from a parent, guardian, bystander or other emergency service professional is invaluable. What was the drug that the child has accidentally ingested, when did it happen, and how many tablets are missing?

"Reading the wreckage" of a road traffic accident will help to predict occult injuries. Why is there a bottle of juice on the back seat, but the baby seat is empty? Has the baby been ejected? Is it under the front seat? Has it been left with a child minder? If it has been ejected, suspect severe injuries irrespective of the vital signs.

Communication is a common failing in scene management. It is important to communicate with other services at the scene. To pull in different directions can only be to the detriment of the patient. It is important to communicate effectively with ambulance control, or directly with the receiving hospital. Experience at the hospital will show that a relayed telephone communication (a "courtesy call") from ambulance control may contain insufficient information to trigger an appropriate response—a direct radio message is of greater use. A standard format to this communication is useful (see Box 4.1).

Box 4.1 THE "ASHICE" FORMAT FOR PRE-HOSPITAL COMMUNICATION

A Age
S Sex
H History
I Injuries/illness found and suspected
C Current condition (vital signs)
E Expected time and mode of arrival (A&E)

Triage

When there are two or more casualties it is essential to prioritise for treatment. To fail to triage may result in resources being diverted to less needy casualties. Evidence shows that triage is done badly. This is because there is a tendency to "eyeball" casualties and prioritise on the injuries that can be seen. Such an "anatomical" method of triage is poorly reproducible between individuals. It also requires patients to be exposed for the injuries to be seen, which is slow and impractical pre-hospital.

The alternative is to assign triage priorities on the consequences of injury, that is to say a change in vital signs (for example, pulse, blood pressure, respiratory rate, and Glasgow Coma Scale). This is "physiological" triage and it is accepted that these methods are simple, rapid, safe, and reproducible. However, when triaging children it is important to use appropriate ranges of vital signs for a particular age. If adult vital signs are used, small children will be over-triaged (given an inappropriately high triage priority). Paediatric triage is discussed in more detail later in Appendix G.

Examples

Consider the following situations. How would you initially manage the incident? These events are all based on actual case histories.

Example 1 An elderly woman is driving her elderly friend to lunch. The driver suffers a cardiac arrest. The car mounts the pavement and strikes a young mother, her 2-year-old child walking on reins, and a 9-month-old baby in a pram. The baby is thrown out of the pram and is lying on the pavement unresponsive, but is breathing spontaneously. The mother is trapped under the car, and loses vital signs shortly after the arrival of the first ambulance. The driver of the car is in fine ventricular fibrillation. The 2-year-old is screaming hysterically, with no visible injuries.

Example 2 A stolen car is involved in a high-speed road traffic accident in the early evening. The male driver and female front seat passenger sustain severe injuries, and there is severe deformation of the vehicle. There is a child seat in the car, and a half-drunk bottle of milk. No baby can be found.

Example 3 A teenage boy at a rave with a 15 000 crowd has taken Ecstasy, atenolol 200 mg (to counter the tachycardia side effect of Ecstasy) and diazepam. He suffers a cardiac arrest in the toilets. The rave continues while the ambulance is called.

Answers

1 Control then ACT!
2 Control then ACT!
3 Control then ACT!

For the management of these casualties, continue reading this book.

Questions

1 How will you prioritise your actions at an incident involving children?
2 Why is it important to remember good scene management at an incident involving children?
3 How many casualties do you need to require triage methods to be used?

5

Transport of children

OBJECTIVES

After reading this chapter you should be able to:

- List the two phases of transportation of children
- List the five elements of the systematic approach to prehospital care
- State where definitive care is best provided

INTRODUCTION

Transportation of children falls within two main categories. Primary transfer involves the child being moved to the initial receiving hospital and secondary transfer is usually between the initial receiving hospital and a specialist (paediatric) treatment centre.

It is important not to delay the patient at the scene unduly, but it is also important that a child is not transferred between hospitals without adequate preparation and planning. Depending on the situation and the patient's condition this may take from minutes to hours.

This chapter therefore focuses on both the out of hospital phases of patient care.

PRE-HOSPITAL TRANSPORTATION

Historically, the provision of pre-hospital paediatric care has been very basic in Britain. The ambulance service has come a long way since the relatively recent days of fairly basic training and low levels of equipment. There are still members of the service who will remember single manning assisted by a friendly police constable to treat and transport seriously ill patients. The treatment relied upon rapid transport to hospital with the minimum of treatment or delay.

The term "**scoop and run**" is still used by ambulance personnel to describe this method of response.

Since the development of ambulance service training in the 1980s and the more recent development of paediatric training for paramedics and pre-hospital doctors, the scope of treatment available in the pre-hospital setting has developed greatly. Drugs and a range of advanced procedures previously only seen within the hospital are now commonly available at the scene of an accident. The term "**stay and play**" has now entered the vocabulary, describing the unnecessarily prolonged treatment of a patient on the scene prior to moving to the hospital.

As the training and treatment options in the pre-hospital setting increase, the provider of pre-hospital care has a wider scope of skills available, but with it comes an increased responsibility for deciding how much treatment to provide before transporting the patient to the hospital.

> **The difficulty for providers of pre-hospital care nowadays is to avoid both "stay and play" and "scoop and run"**

With these developments in pre-hospital skills and training, some may be under the illusion that patients can and should be fully stabilised before leaving the scene of an incident. Unfortunately, there are increasing reports of patients who have been provided with prolonged treatment at the scene which has failed to increase their long term survival.

It should always be remembered that **definitive care can only be provided within the hospital**. A systematic approach (summarised in Box 5.1) must be employed in the pre-hospital setting to assess the child's condition and whether to treat on the scene or move to hospital without delay.

> **Box 5.1   SYSTEMATIC APPROACH TO PRE-HOSPITAL PATIENT CARE**
>
> ● Primary assessment
> ● Resuscitation
> ● Secondary assessment
> ● Emergency treatment
> ● Definitive care

Primary assessment

A primary assessment that follows the established ABCD principles should be undertaken to establish if any immediately life threatening conditions are present. If any are found, consider moving the child to hospital urgently, only delaying to undertake immediate life saving procedures which cannot be undertaken while travelling to hospital. There are, in fact, few procedures that must be administered prior to moving a sick child, and these are fully covered in the text of this manual.

Airway management or ventilation is obviously appropriate on the scene, while intravenous access (in a patient who is not trapped) can be a common cause of delay, and should ideally be done during transport. If the child has an internal bleed remember that the treatment is surgery and any delay in getting the child to the operating table will reduce the chance of survival.

Secondary assessment

If no life threatening conditions are found then a brief secondary survey may be undertaken, preferably in the warm environment of the ambulance. This secondary survey must not delay transportation without justification, or cause distress to the child. If any life threatening problems are found during this survey, it must be abandoned, the problem dealt with, and the patient transported urgently to hospital.

Monitoring

During transportation to hospital any appropriate procedures such as intravenous cannulation/intraosseous infusion etc should be initiated. The ABCs must be continuously assessed and any relevant monitoring equipment connected to the patient.

The patient should be transported promptly and safely to hospital in a manner that does not cause unnecessary discomfort to the patient or transporting staff.

Communications

The receiving hospital must be alerted as soon as is practicable and all relevant information passed in a clear manner (see Box 4.1). The information passed to the receiving hospital should include no less than:

- The child's age.
- Condition/type of injuries.
- Treatment initiated.
- Expected time of arrival.
- Contact code for crew.

Many teams of specialist staff may be involved in the treatment of a seriously ill child and must be given time to prepare personnel and resources to be available for the arrival of the child. It is very common for receiving hospitals not to be alerted, resulting in unjustifiable delays in the treatment of the child on arrival at hospital.

Communication with the receiving hospital must be treated as an integral part of the child's treatment in the same manner as the primary or secondary assessment. The aim is to provide seamless treatment between the pre-hospital and hospital settings, resulting in the best possible provision of care to the patient.

Some may interpret this approach to the transportation of children as a return to the old "scoop and run" method of treatment. The essential difference is that the treatment is based on an informed assessment of the patient's condition, immediate life saving procedures are initiated without inappropriate delays, and the receiving hospital is prepared for accepting and continuing the treatment of the patient.

> **The answer to the question, "Do we scoop and run or stay and play?" is "neither!"**

INTER-HOSPITAL TRANSFER

Sick or injured children may initially be taken to a unit which can resuscitate or stabilise but may be unable to offer further acute or longer term medical management. Such children will subsequently be transferred to another hospital or department.

It is essential to evaluate, resuscitate, and stabilise the child's condition prior to transfer to a more specialised unit.

Whatever the injury or illness the airway must be secured and ventilation must be adequate. Intravenous access must be established and fluids and/or life saving drugs given. Proper evaluation requires a thorough examination to show whether any orthopaedic, surgical or medical procedures should be carried out prior to transportation. Baseline haematological and biochemical samples should be taken when the intravenous lines are placed and essential imaging should be carried out at this time.

The staff at the receiving hospital or department must be contacted prior to arranging transport. They must be clearly told what has happened, the state of the child, the treatment received, and what transport facilities and staff are needed. Both teams can then decide if the child is stable enough for transport and whether the referring or receiving hospital will provide the staff to supervise transfer. Joint management by the referring hospital and transport team should commence immediately since successful initial resuscitation and stabilisation is crucial to the ultimate outcome. It must be stressed that this initial role is, and must remain, the responsibility of the referring unit and should be provided at a senior level in conjunction with service given by the receiving hospital staff.

Mode of transfer

Transfer of patients in the UK is usually undertaken by road ambulance. As more Services and Trusts merge and expand, the facility to transport patients by air has become an increasingly common option. When deciding on the most appropriate method of transfer, staff should bear in mind the potential difficulties that may arise:

- **Road ambulance**—readily available, has adequate space, and costs relatively little.
- **Helicopter**—quicker than road ambulance, readily available (Ambulance Trusts, police or RAF/Navy) but have problems with lack of space, noise and vibration, which may make monitoring difficult. They are also expensive.

For transfer over very long distances (for example, country to country), fixed wing aircraft can be used.

Equipment

Dedicated transport equipment for monitoring and therapy should be available in the emergency department. Familiarity with such equipment is a prerequisite for all emergency staff who are involved in the transport of a critically ill child. A list of essential equipment is shown in Box 5.2.

Box 5.2 PAEDIATRIC RESUSCITATION EQUIPMENT

- **Airway**

  1 Oropharyngeal airway sizes 000, 00, 0, 1, 2, 3
  2 Endotracheal tubes sizes 2.5–7.5 mm uncuffed (in 0.5 mm steps) and 7.5 mm cuffed
  3 Laryngoscopes:

     - straight paediatric blades
     - adult curved blade

  4 Magill forceps
  5 Yankauer sucker
  6 Soft suction catheters
  7 Needle cricothyroidotomy set

- **Breathing**

  1 Oxygen masks with reservoir
  2 Self-inflating bags (with reservoir)

     - 240 ml infant size
     - 500 ml child size
     - 1600 ml adult size

  3 Face masks

     - infant: circular 01, 1, 2
     - child: anatomical 2, 3
     - adult: anatomical 4, 5

  4 Catheter mount and connectors
  5 Ayre's T-piece

- **Circulation**

  1 ECG monitor defibrillator (with paediatric paddles)
  2 Non-invasive blood pressure monitor (with infant and child sized cuffs)
  3 Pulse oximeter (with infant and child sized probes)

4 Intravenous access requirements

   - Intravenous cannulae (as available) 18–25 g
   - Intraosseous infusion needles 16–18 g
   - Graduated burette
   - Intravenous giving sets
   - Syringes 1–50 ml

5 Intravenous drip monitoring device
6 Cut down set

- **Fluids**

   - 0.9% saline
   - Hartmann's solution or Ringer's lactate
   - 4% dextrose and 0.18% saline
   - 5% dextrose
   - Colloid
   - 4.5% Human albumin solution

- **Drugs**

   - Adrenaline (epinephrine) 1:10 000
   - Adrenaline 1:1000
   - Atropine 0.6 or 1 mg/ml
   - Sodium bicarbonate 8.4% + 4.2%
   - Dopamine 40 mg/ml
   - Lignocaine (lidocaine) 1%
   - Dextrose 10% and 25%
   - Calcium chloride 10%
   - Frusemide 20 mg/ml
   - Mannitol 10% or 20%
   - Antibiotics: penicillin, chloramphenicol, gentamicin, ampicillin, ceftazidime, cefotaxime

- **Miscellaneous**

   - Stick test for glucose
   - Chest drain set

The transfer

Airway and Breathing

The airway should be adequately secured and intubated patients ventilated mechanically rather than manually to allow other procedures to be undertaken if required. Some ambulance ventilators only have settings for adults, therefore if it is intended to use the ambulance equipment confirm its suitability prior to loading the child.

Modern portable suction allows for adequate tracheal toilet to be carried out and will reduce the chances of tube blockage.

It is vital that appropriate sedative agents, together with muscle relaxants, are administered for the comfort and safety of all intubated children during the transfer. These agents reduce the risk of accidental extubation (reintubating in the less than ideal confines of an ambulance may be extremely difficult). Provided there are no contraindications (such as suspected fractured base of skull), nasal tubes are generally easier to fix in place and less liable to fall out. The attending doctor must be completely happy to re-intubate the child in the unfortunate event of accidental extubation.

Circulation

Battery powered syringe pumps capable of holding syringes up to 50 ml are indispensable during the transfer. Patients with established or potential haemodynamic instability may have numerous catheters, central, and peripheral lines *in situ* and extreme care must be taken when lifting the child into the ambulance. This is a common time for accidental displacement of lines that may be needed for rapid administration of drugs or fluids.

Disability

The transfer of the comatose child requires consideration, especially in the context of head injuries. Coma is the sign of significant "brain failure" and requires emergency treatment to prevent secondary central nervous system damage. Full assessment and initial management of ABC and seizures take precedence over the need to get the patient to the CT or MRI scanner.

Exposure

Children become cold very quickly, particularly if seriously ill. Adequate steps must be taken to ensure that hypothermia does not occur. Blankets or duvets should cover all exposed parts and all infused fluids should be warmed, if possible.

Documentation

All procedures should be documented. The child's notes, radiographs, charts, and any cross-matched blood should be taken to the receiving unit. Results of investigations that become available after the child has left should be communicated to the receiving unit immediately. A communication system with the referring hospital should be agreed.

Parents

Try to keep parents with the child whenever possible. When parents use their own transport make sure they travel either before or some minutes after the ambulance. Don't allow them to "tailgate" the vehicle as an accident may result. It is also important to confirm they know the location of the receiving hospital prior to letting them leave.

CHECKLIST PRIOR TO TRANSPORTING A CHILD BETWEEN HOSPITALS

1 Is the airway protected and ventilation satisfactory? (substantiated by blood gases, pH and pulse oximetry if possible)
2 Is the neck properly immobilised?
3 Is there sufficient oxygen available for the journey?
4 Is vascular access secure and will the pumps in use during transport work by battery?
5 Have adequate fluids been given prior to transport?
6 Are fractured limbs appropriately splinted and immobilised?
7 Are appropriate monitors in use? Are they compatible with the ambulance electrical system?
8 Will the child/baby be sufficiently warm during the journey?
9 Is documentation available? Include:

> Child's name
> Age
> Date of birth
> Weight
> Radiographs taken
> Clinical notes
> Observation charts
> Neurological observation chart
> The time and route of all drugs given
> Fluid charts
> Ventilator records
> Results of investigations

10 Has the case been discussed with the receiving team directly?
11 Have plans been discussed with the parents?

SUMMARY

Meticulous attention to initial assessment and resuscitation together with appropriate emergency treatment will reduce the chance of transport related morbidity and mortality. Critically ill and injured children can be transferred by a specialised paediatric transport team with minimal related complications.

Questions

1 List the five elements of pre-hospital patient care.
2 Where is the definitive care provided best?

PART II

LIFE SUPPORT

6

Basic life support

> **OBJECTIVES**
>
> After reading this chapter you should be able to:
>
> - Describe the steps required to safely approach and assess a collapsed infant and child
> - Identify the appropriate resuscitation techniques to adopt for all ages of children
> - Describe the assessment and treatment of a child and infant with an airway obstruction

INTRODUCTION

Paediatric basic life support (BLS) is not simply a scaled down version of that provided for adults. As discussed in Chapters 1 and 2 of this manual, the pathways leading to cardiorespiratory arrest are rarely due to primary cardiac disease as in adults, and the anatomy and physiology are also different. When resuscitating children, oxygen delivery rather than defibrillation is the critical step, as ventricular fibrillation is rare. Resuscitation techniques also need to reflect the anatomy and physiology of the different age groups.

Although the general principles of paediatric resuscitation are the same as for adults, the exact techniques employed need to be varied according to the size of the child. A somewhat artificial distinction is therefore made between:

- Infants (less than 1 year old).
- Small children (aged 1–8 years).
- Older children (aged over 8 years).

By applying the basic techniques described, a single rescuer can support the vital respiratory and circulatory functions of a collapsed child, with no equipment.

Basic life support is the foundation on which advanced life support is built. Therefore it is essential that all advanced life support providers are proficient at basic techniques and that they are capable of ensuring that basic life support is provided correctly and continuously during resuscitation.

ASSESSMENT AND TREATMENT

Once the child has been approached safely and a simple test for responsiveness has been carried out, assessment and treatment of the airway, breathing, and circulation is undertaken. The overall sequence of basic life support in paediatric cardiopulmonary arrest is summarised in Figure 6.1.

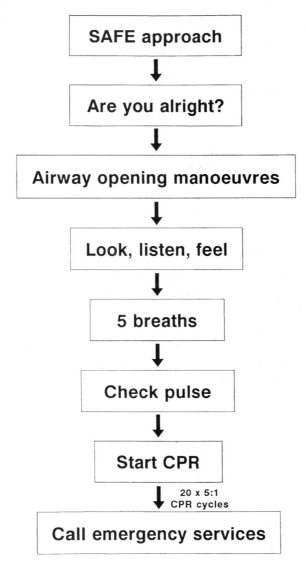

Figure 6.1. The overall sequence of basic life support in cardiopulmonary arrest (CPR = cardiopulmonary resuscitation)

The SAFE approach

Additional help should be summoned rapidly. Furthermore, it is essential that the rescuer does not become a second victim, and that the child is removed from continuing danger as quickly as possible. These considerations should precede an assessment of the victim. They are summarised in Figure 6.2.

Are you alright?

The initial simple assessment of responsiveness consists of asking the child "Are you alright?", and *gently* shaking him or her by the shoulders. Infants and very small children who cannot talk yet, and older children who are very scared are unlikely to reply meaningfully, but may make some sound or open their eyes to the rescuer's voice.

In cases associated with trauma, children and infants must not be shaken.

S hout for help

A pproach with care

F ree from danger

E valuate ABC

Figure 6.2. The SAFE approach

Airway-opening manoeuvres

An obstructed airway may be the primary problem, and correction of the obstruction can result in recovery without further intervention.

If a child is having difficulty breathing, but is conscious, then transport to hospital should be arranged as quickly as possible. A child will often find the best position to maintain his or her own airway, and should not be forced to adopt a position which they find less comfortable. Attempts to improve a partially maintained airway in an environment where immediate advanced support is not available can be dangerous, since total obstruction may occur.

If the child is not breathing, the airway may have been blocked by the tongue falling back to obstruct the pharynx. An attempt to open the airway should be made using the head tilt/chin lift manoeuvre. The rescuer places the hand nearest to the child's head on the forehead, and applies pressure to tilt the head back gently. The fingers of the other hand should then be placed at the point of the chin and the chin lifted upwards. Care should be taken not to press on the soft tissue of the airway. As this action can close the child's mouth, it may be necessary to use the thumb of the same hand to part the lips slightly.

The desirable degrees of tilt are: *neutral* in the infant and *sniffing* in the child, as shown in Figures 6.3 and 6.4.

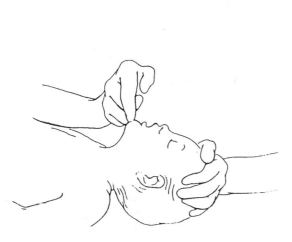

Figure 6.3. Neutral position in an infant

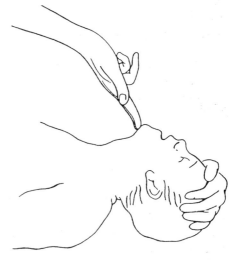

Figure 6.4. Sniffing position in a child

If there is a history of trauma, the head tilt/chin lift manoeuvre may exacerbate cervical spine injury. The safest airway intervention in these circumstances is the use of a jaw thrust (Figure 6.5). This is achieved by placing two or three fingers under the angle of the mandible bilaterally, and lifting the jaw upwards. This technique may be made easier if the rescuer's elbows are resting on the same surface as the child is lying.

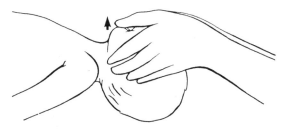

Figure 6.5. Jaw thrust

The finger sweep technique should not be used in children. The soft palate is easily damaged and bleeding from within the mouth can worsen the situation. Furthermore, foreign bodies may be forced further down the airway; they can become lodged below the vocal cords (vocal folds) and become more difficult to remove.

If a foreign body is not obvious, inspection should be made under direct vision and, if appropriate, removed using Magill's forceps.

Look, Listen, Feel

While maintaining an airway-opening manoeuvre, the patency of the airway should then be assessed. This is achieved by:

- **LOOK**ing for chest movement
- **LISTEN**ing at the child's mouth and nose for breath sounds
- **FEEL**ing with your cheek for air movement

and is best achieved by the rescuer placing his or her face above the child's face, with the ear over the nose, the cheek over the mouth, and the eyes looking along the line of the chest. Look, listen and feel for breathing for up to 10 seconds before deciding that breathing is absent.

If the child's chest and abdomen are moving but no airflow can be detected, the airway is obstructed. Readjust the airway and consider obstruction by a foreign body.

Five breaths

If the airway opening techniques described above do not result in the resumption of breathing, exhaled air resuscitation should be commenced.

While the airway is kept open as described above, the rescuer breathes in and seals his or her mouth around the victim's mouth, or mouth and nose, as shown in Figure 6.6. The rescuer then breathes out watching for the chest of the infant/child to rise. If the mouth alone is used, the nose should be pinched closed using the thumb and index fingers of the hand that is maintaining the head tilt. Slow exhalation of 1–1.5 seconds by the rescuer should result in the victim's chest rising while reducing the chance of gastric distension. Once the chest has risen, the rescuer's mouth is removed from the child/infant and the chest observed to fall.

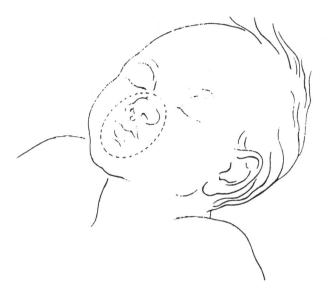

Figure 6.6. Mouth to mouth-and-nose (infant)

Five initial rescue breaths should be attempted.

> **Box 6.1 GENERAL GUIDANCE FOR EXHALED AIR RESUSCITATION**
> * The chest should be seen to rise
> * Inflation pressure may be higher since airways are small
> * Slow breaths at the lowest pressure reduce gastric distension

As children vary in size, only general guidance can be given regarding the volume and pressure of inflation. At least two of the five initial breaths should cause the chest to rise. If the chest does not rise then the airway is not clear. The usual cause is failure to apply correctly the airway-opening techniques discussed above. Readjust the head tilt/chin lift position, and attempt a further five breaths.

Failure of both head tilt/chin lift and jaw thrust should lead to the suspicion that a foreign body is causing the obstruction, and the appropriate action should be taken (see below).

Check pulse

Once the initial five breaths have been given as above, attention should be turned to the circulation.

Assessment

Inadequacy of the circulation is recognised by the absence of a central pulse for 10 seconds or by the presence of a pulse at an insufficient rate. In children, as in adults, the carotid artery in the neck can be palpated.

In infants the neck is generally short and fat, and the carotid artery may be difficult to identify. Therefore the brachial artery in the medial aspect of the antecubital fossa (Figure 6.7), or the femoral artery in the groin, should be felt.

Any movement, including swallowing or breathing (other than an occasional gasp), should be noted during the diagnosis of cardiac arrest.

If the pulse is present and at an adequate rate, but apnoea persists, exhaled air resuscitation must be continued at a rate of 20 breaths per minute, until spontaneous breathing resumes.

33

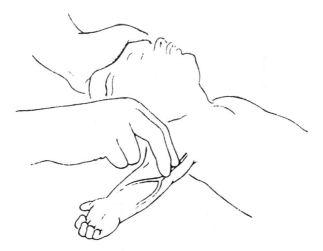

Figure 6.7. Feeling the brachial pulse

Start CPR

If the pulse is absent for 10 seconds or inadequate (less than 60 beats per minute in infants) or you are unsure, cardiac compressions combined with breathing should be initiated.

Cardiac compression

For the best output the child must be placed lying flat on his or her back, on a hard surface. In infants it is said that the palm of the rescuer's hand can be used for this purpose, but this may prove difficult in practice.

Children vary in size, and the exact nature of the compressions given should reflect this. In general, infants (less than 1 year) require a different technique from small children. In children over 8 years of age, the method used in adults can be applied with appropriate modifications for their size.

The depth of compressions can be estimated at one-third of the depth of the chest for infants and children. The rate of compressions is 100 per minute for infants and children.

Infants   As the infant heart is lower in relation to external landmarks when compared to older children and adults, the area of compression is found by imagining a line between the nipples and compressing over the sternum one finger-breadth below this line. Two fingers are used to compress the chest. This is shown in Figure 6.8. Alternatively infant cardiac compression can be achieved using the hand-encircling technique: the infant is held with both the rescuer's hands encircling the chest. The thumbs are placed over the correct part of the sternum (see above) and compression carried out, as shown in Figure 6.9.

Small children   The area of compression is one finger-breadth above the xiphisternum. The heel of one hand is used to depress the sternum (Figure 6.10).

Larger children   The area of compression is two finger-breadths above the xiphisternum. The heels of both hands are used to depress the sternum one-third of the depth of the chest (Figure 6.11).

Once the correct technique has been chosen and the area for compression identified, five compressions should be given.

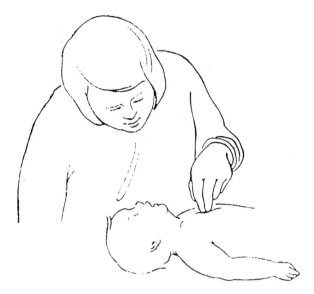

Figure 6.8. Infant chest compression: two-finger technique

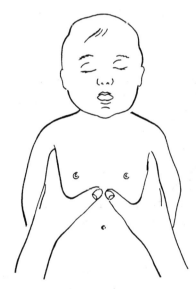

Figure 6.9. Infant chest compression: hand encircling technique

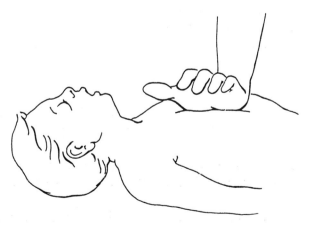

Figure 6.10. Chest compression in small children

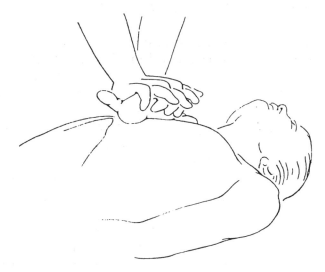

Figure 6.11. Chest compression in older children

Continuing CPR

A ratio of five compressions to one ventilation is maintained whatever the number of rescuers in infants and small children. For children over the age of 8 years, a two-handed method of chest compression can be used with a ratio of 15 compressions to two ventilations for a single rescuer and five compressions to one ventilation for two rescuers.

Call emergency services

If no help has arrived, the emergency services must be contacted after approximately 20 full cardiopulmonary resuscitation cycles have been delivered (ie 1 minute). Apart from this interruption to summon help, basic life support must not be interrupted unless the child moves or takes a breath.

The cardiopulmonary resuscitation manoeuvres recommended for infants and children are summarised in Table 6.1.

Table 6.1. Summary of basic life support techniques in infants and children

	Infant (<1 year)	Small child (1–8 years)	Larger child (over 8 years)
Airway			
Head tilt position	Neutral	Sniffing	Sniffing
Breathing			
Initial slow breaths	5	5	5
Circulation			
Pulse check	Brachial or femoral	Carotid	Carotid
Landmark	One finger-breadth below nipple line	One finger-breadth above xiphisternum	Two finger-breadths above xiphisternum
Technique	Two fingers or encircling	One hand	Two hands
Cardiopulmonary resuscitation			
Ratio	5:1	5:1	5:1 (15:2)
Cycles per minute	20	20	20 (4)

BASIC LIFE SUPPORT AND INFECTION RISK

There have been a few reports of transmission of infectious diseases from casualties to rescuers during mouth-to-mouth resuscitation. The most serious concern in children is meningococcus, and rescuers involved in the resuscitation of the airway in such patients should take standard prophylactic antibiotics (usually rifampicin).

There have been no reported cases of transmission of either hepatitis B or human immunodeficiency virus (HIV) through mouth-to-mouth ventilation. Blood-to-blood contact is the single most important route of transmission of these viruses, and in non-trauma resuscitations the risks are negligible. Sputum, saliva, sweat, tears, urine, and vomit are low risk fluids. Precautions should be taken if possible in cases where there might be contact with blood, semen, vaginal secretions, cerebrospinal fluid, pleural and peritoneal fluids, and amniotic fluid. Precautions are also recommended if any bodily secretion contains visible blood. Devices which prevent direct contact between the rescuer and the victim (such as resuscitation masks) can be used to lower risk; gauze swabs or any other porous material placed over the victim's mouth are of no benefit in this regard.

The number of children in the UK with AIDS or HIV-1 infection in June 1992 was estimated at 501, while the number of adults similarly affected was estimated at 23806 (a ratio of 1:47). If transmission of HIV-1 does occur it is therefore much more likely to be from adult rescuer to child rather than the other way around.

Although practice manikins have not been shown to be a source of infection, regular cleaning is recommended, and should be carried out as shown in the manufacturer's instructions.

THE CHOKING CHILD

Introduction

The vast majority of deaths from foreign body aspiration occur in pre-school children. Virtually anything may be inhaled. The diagnosis is very rarely clear-cut, but should be suspected if the onset of respiratory compromise is sudden and is associated with coughing, gagging, and stridor. Airway obstruction may also occur with infections such as acute epiglottitis and croup. In such cases attempts to relieve the obstruction using the methods described below are dangerous. Children with known or suspected infectious causes of obstruction, and those who are still breathing and in whom the cause of obstruction is unclear, should be taken to hospital urgently.

The physical methods of clearing the airway, described below, should therefore only be performed if:

1 The diagnosis of foreign body aspiration is clear-cut, and apnoea has occurred.
2 Head tilt/chin lift and jaw thrust have failed to enable ventilation of an apnoeic child. The sequence of instructions is shown in Figure 6.12.

Infants

Abdominal thrusts may cause intra-abdominal injury in infants. Therefore a combination of back blows and chest thrusts is recommended for the relief of foreign body obstruction in this age group.

The baby is placed along one of the rescuer's arms in a head-down position. The rescuer then rests his or her arm along the thigh, and delivers five back blows with the heel of the free hand.

If the obstruction is not relieved the baby is turned over and laid along the rescuer's thigh, still in a head-down position. Five chest thrusts are given—using the same

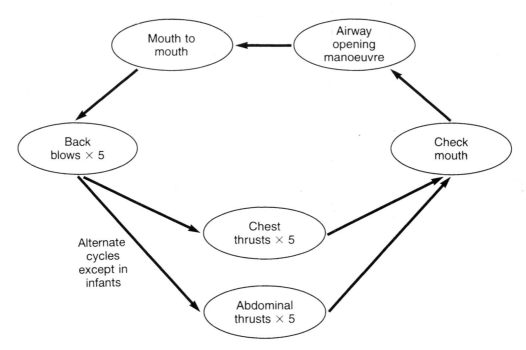

Figure 6.12. Clearing the airway

landmarks as for cardiac compression but slower. If an infant is too large to allow the single-arm technique described above to be used, then the same manoeuvres can be performed by lying the baby across the rescuer's lap. These techniques are shown in Figures 6.13 and 6.14.

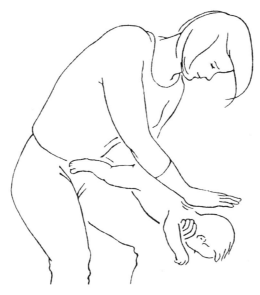

Figure 6.13. Back blows in an infant

If five back blows followed by five chest thrusts fail to remove a foreign body, check the mouth and remove any visible obstruction. Attempt to open the airway using the head tilt/chin lift or jaw thrust manoeuvre and then reassess breathing. If the infant is not breathing, attempt five rescue breaths. If the airway is still obstructed, repeat this sequence until the infant breathes spontaneously (see Figure 6.12).

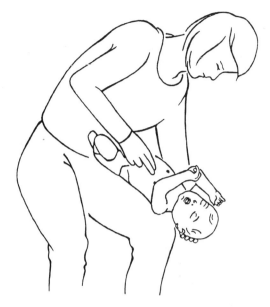

Figure 6.14. Chest thrusts in an infant

Children

Back blows can be used as in infants (see Figure 6.15). In the older child the Heimlich manoeuvre (abdominal thrust) can also be used. As in the adult, this can be performed with the victim standing, sitting, kneeling, or lying.

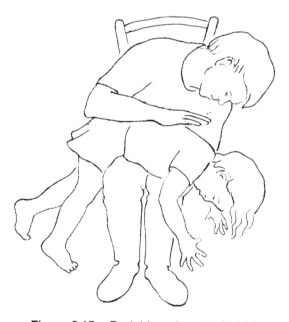

Figure 6.15. Back blows in a small child

If this is to be attempted with the child standing, kneeling, or sitting, the rescuer moves behind the victim and passes his or her arms around the victim's body. Owing to the height of children, it may be necessary for an adult to stand the child on a box or other convenient object to carry out the standing manoeuvre effectively. One hand is formed into a fist and placed against the child's abdomen above the umbilicus and below the xiphisternum. The other hand is placed over the fist, and both hands are thrust sharply upwards into the abdomen. This is repeated five times unless the object causing the obstruction is expelled before then. This technique is shown in Figure 6.16.

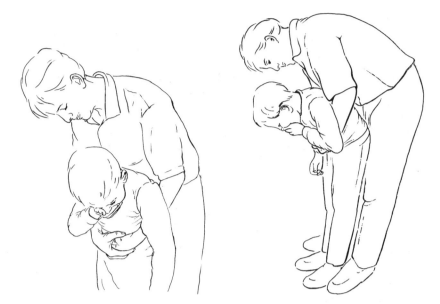

Figure 6.16. The Heimlich manoeuvre

If five back blows followed by five chest thrusts fail to remove a foreign body, check the mouth and remove any visible obstruction. Attempt to open the airway using the head tilt/chin lift or jaw thrust manoeuvre and then reassess breathing. If the child is not breathing, attempt five rescue breaths. If the airway is still obstructed repeat this sequence, alternating between chest thrusts and abdominal thrusts until the child breathes spontaneously (see Figure 6.12).

To carry out abdominal thrusts in a supine child, the rescuer kneels at his or her feet (Figure 6.17). If the child is large, it may be necessary to kneel astride him or her. The heel of one hand is placed against the child's abdomen above the umbilicus and below the xiphisternum. The other hand is placed on top of the first, and both hands are thrust sharply upwards into the abdomen with care being taken to direct the thrust in the midline. This is repeated five times unless the object causing the obstruction is expelled before then.

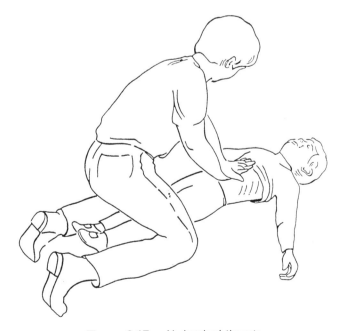

Figure 6.17. Abdominal thrusts

SUMMARY

- The SAFE approach should be used when approaching all collapsed children.
- Assessment and treatment follows the ABC sequence.
- Although the general principles are the same, specific basic life support techniques need to be employed for infants, small children, and older children.
- The sequence for removal of an airway obstruction for children includes back blows, chest thrusts and abdominal thrusts, depending on the age of the child.

Questions

1 What do the letters of the SAFE approach represent?
2 What is the recommended head position to achieve when performing a head tilt and chin lift on:

   (a) an infant?
   (b) a small child?

3 What manoeuvres are recommended when attempting to clear an obstructed airway from:

   (a) an infant?
   (b) a child?

7

Advanced support of the airway and ventilation

OBJECTIVES

After reading this chapter you should be able to:

● Select appropriately sized airway equipment for different aged children
● Describe the different methods of maintaining the airway and adequate ventilation

---

INTRODUCTION

Management of airway and breathing has priority in the resuscitation of patients of all ages; the rate at which respiratory function can deteriorate in children is particularly rapid. It is vital that effective resuscitation techniques can be applied quickly and in order of priority. To do so, it is useful to appreciate the differences between adults and children, and essential to be familiar with commonly used equipment. Techniques for obtaining a patent and protected airway, and of achieving adequate ventilation and oxygenation, must be learned and practised. Finally, these techniques must be integrated into a prioritised system of care, planned in advance, to avoid delays and uncertainties in emergency situations.

EQUIPMENT FOR MANAGING THE AIRWAY

The airway equipment indicated in Box 7.1 should be readily available. It is crucial that familiarity with it is gained before it is needed in an emergency situation.

Box 7.1 AIRWAY EQUIPMENT

● Suction devices
● Pharyngeal airways
● Laryngoscopes
● Endotracheal tubes, introducers and connectors
● Magill forceps
● Tracheal suction catheters

Suction devices

In the field, hand-powered or foot-operated suction apparatus is convenient and reliable, although the mechanism of action creates an intermittent suction effect and requires movement and physical effort on the part of the operator. Vacuum canisters provide an effective alternative but become useless when discharged. Battery-powered devices may be heavy and less reliable than manual ones, although they are versatile in the pre-hospital setting. In the ambulance, other sources of power are available. Electrical suction devices may be used on the vehicle's 12 volt dc supply or, if a power inverter is provided, may run on a 240 volt ac supply. Oxygen-powered suckers are commonly used but it should be remembered that frequent use may deplete oxygen stores required for mechanical ventilation.

Hand-powered suckers often have wide tubing, which may fill the mouth of a small child. Smaller tubing or an alternative ending can be attached but may convert the sucker into a two-handed device and limit the ability to remove vomit. Mucus extractors are a simple option in neonates. Endobronchial catheters can be attached to suction devices to aspirate down an endotracheal tube after intubation. The Yankauer sucker ending remains the standard to be used in conjunction with electrical or gas powered devices in the ambulance. It is available in both adult and paediatric sizes. The paediatric size has a side hole which can be occluded by a finger or thumb, allowing control over vacuum pressure.

The arrangements for suction in the field are a compromise between power, control, and portability. The pre-hospital carer should be familiar with the idiosyncrasies of each method (Table 7.1).

Table 7.1. Suction devices

Power source for suction device	Problem
Oxygen	Less oxygen available for patient
Gas canister	Useless when discharged
Electrical	Batteries must be kept charged
Manual	Coordination between foot pumping and suction is a skill which needs practice

Pharyngeal airways

There are three main types of pharyngeal airway:

● Oropharyngeal.
● Nasopharyngeal.
● Laryngeal mask.

The oropharyngeal or Guedel airway is used in the obtunded patient to provide a patent airway channel between the tongue and the posterior pharyngeal wall. It may also be used to stabilise the position of an oral endotracheal tube. In the awake patient with an intact gag reflex, it may not be tolerated and may provoke vomiting. It is available in a variety of sizes. A suitably sized airway reaches from the centre of the incisors to the angle of the mandible when laid on the face concave side up. An inappropriate size may cause laryngospasm, mucosal trauma or may worsen the airway obstruction. Two techniques for insertion are described in Chapter 14.

The nasopharyngeal airway is often better tolerated than the Guedel airway. It is contraindicated in fractures of the anterior base of the skull. It may also cause significant haemorrhage from the friable, vascular, nasal mucosa. A suitable length can be estimated by measuring from the tip of the nose to the tragus of the ear. An appropriate diameter is one that just fits into the nostril without causing sustained blanching of the alae nasai. As small-sized nasopharyngeal airways are not commercially available, shortened endotracheal tubes may be used.

The laryngeal mask has been referred to as a cuffed, self-retaining oropharyngeal airway. It has gained widespread use in general anaesthesia and is a useful alternative airway, especially when intubation is difficult or impossible, or if access to the patient is limited. It connects conveniently to a self-inflating bag. While the laryngeal mask airway (LMA) (Figure 7.1) sits over the larynx, preventing some of the upper airway secretions from coming into contact with the larynx, it by no means protects the tracheobronchial tree against aspiration.

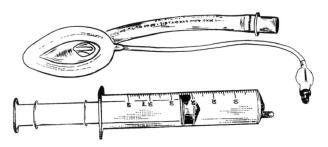

Figure 7.1   Picture of laryngeal mask airway

Sizing is estimated by following the recommendations in Table 7.2.

Table 7.2.   Sizing of laryngeal mask airways

Laryngeal mask airway size	Size of child	Volume of air to inflate cuff
1	Neonate–6 kg	4 ml
2	6.5–20 kg	10 ml
$2\frac{1}{2}$	20–30 kg	14 ml
3	30–small adult	20 ml
4	Normal adult	30 ml
5	Large adult	40 ml

Laryngoscopes

There are two principal designs of laryngoscope for use in children: straight-bladed and curved-bladed. In general, the straight-bladed laryngoscope is designed to lift the epiglottis under the tip of the blade, whereas the curved-blade laryngoscope is designed to rest in the vallecula. The straight-bladed device can also be placed short of the epiglottis in the vallecula. The advantage of taking the epiglottis is that it cannot then obscure the view of the vocal cords (vocal folds). The advantage of stopping short of the epiglottis is that it causes less stimulation, and is less likely to cause laryngospasm. The blade length should be varied according to the age. It should be noted that it is possible to intubate successfully with a blade that is too long, but not with one that is too short. In general, straight blades are preferred up to the age of 1 year, and many prefer to use them up to the age of 5 years.

It is important to have a spare laryngoscope available, together with spare bulbs and batteries, to overcome equipment failure. In fibreoptic designs, the bulbs are set in the top of the blade handle rather than in the blade itself. This has advantages in terms of bulb protection and the ability to clean the blade after use.

The essential parts of these laryngoscopes are shown in Figures 7.2 and 7.3. The blade is designed to displace the tongue to the left in order to optimise the view of the larynx. Failure to control the tongue adequately in the haste to see the vocal cords may leave a portion of the tongue overhanging the blade. It may still be possible to see the larynx at first, but as soon as the endotracheal tube is placed into the mouth, the view is obscured.

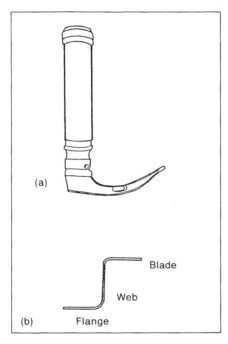

Figure 7.2. (a) Mackintosh curved-blade laryngoscope: (b) blade cross section

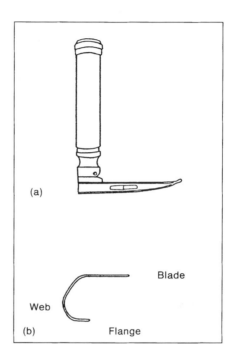

Figure 7.3. (a) Straight-blade laryngoscope; (b) blade cross section

Endotracheal tubes

Endotracheal tubes come in a variety of designs but the plain plastic tube is the most useful in resuscitation. Uncuffed tubes are preferred up until puberty so as not to cause oedema at the cricoid ring.

Estimating the appropriate size of an endotracheal tube is carried out as follows:

Internal diameter (mm) = (age in years/4) + 4
Length (cm) = (age in years/2) + 12 for an oral tube
Length (cm) = (age in years/2) + 15 for a nasal tube

These formulae are appropriate for ages over 1 year. Neonates usually require a tube of internal diameter 3–3.5 mm, although pre-term infants may need a 2.5 mm. Another useful guideline is to use a tube of about the same diameter as the child's little finger, or of such a size that will just fit into the nostril. This also applies to nasopharyngeal airways.

Endotracheal tube introducers

A difficult intubation can be facilitated by the use of a stylet or introducer, placed through the lumen of the endotracheal tube. These are of two types: soft and flexible or firm and malleable. The former can be allowed to project out of the tip of the tube, as long as it is handled very gently. The latter is used to alter the shape of the tube, but can easily damage the tissues if allowed to protrude from the end.

Endotracheal tube connectors

In adults, the proximal end of the tube connectors is of standard size, based on the 15–22 mm system, ensuring that they can be connected to a standard self-inflating bag. The same standard Portex system exists for children, including neonates. However, many prefer to use smaller connectors in infants. The Minilink system is based on diameters of 8.5 mm. Either system works well, but a resuscitation kit containing both can be confusing and dangerous. It is important that a clear decision between these is made so as to avoid this problem.

Magill's forceps

Magill's forceps are used to grasp an endotracheal tube, particularly one inserted through the nose, and pass it through the vocal cords. They are also suitable for removing foreign bodies in the upper airways under direct vision, and are designed to pass into the mouth with the handle at an angle so as not to obscure the view. Magill's forceps are available in both adult and child sizes.

Tracheal suction catheters

These may be required after intubation to remove bronchial secretions or aspirated fluids. In general, the appropriate size in French gauge is numerically twice the internal diameter in millimetres, eg for an endotracheal tube size 3.0 mm the correct suction catheter is a French gauge 6.

Cricothyroidotomy cannulae and ventilation systems

Purpose-made cricothyroidotomy cannulae are available, usually in three sizes: 12 G for an adult, 14 G for a child, and 18 G for a baby. They are less liable to kinking than intravenous cannulae and have a flange for suturing or securing to the neck.

In an emergency a 14 G intravenous cannula can be inserted through the cricothyroid membrane, and oxygen insufflated at 2 l/min to provide some oxygenation (but no ventilation). A side hole can be cut in the oxygen tubing or a Y-connector can be placed between the cannula and the oxygen supply, to allow intermittent occlusion and achieve partial ventilation.

EQUIPMENT FOR PROVIDING OXYGEN AND VENTILATION

The equipment for oxygenation and ventilation indicated in Box 7.2 should be readily available.

Box 7.2 EQUIPMENT FOR OXYGENATION AND VENTILATION

Oxygen source and masks for spontaneous breathing
Face masks (for artificial ventilation)
Self-inflating bags
Mechanical ventilators
Chest tubes
Gastric tubes

Oxygen source and masks for spontaneous breathing

Oxygen cylinders should have an attached flowmeter capable of delivering 15 l/min. A mask with a reservoir bag should be used to provide high concentration oxygen.

Nasal prongs may sometimes be accepted by a child who will not tolerate a mask, but they dry the airway, cause nasal obstruction in infants, and provide an unreliable oxygen concentration. Although the pre-term infant is vulnerable to retrolental fibroplasia associated with high concentration oxygen, high concentrations should never be withheld for immediate resuscitation.

Face masks (for artificial ventilation)

Face masks for mouth-to-mask or bag-valve-mask ventilation in infants are of two main designs. Some masks conform to the anatomy of the child's face and have a low dead space. Circular soft plastic masks give an excellent seal and are preferred by many. Children's masks should be clear to allow the child's colour or the presence of vomit to be seen.

A Laerdal pocket mask is a single-size clear plastic mask with an air-filled cushion rim designed for mouth-to-mask resuscitation. It can be supplied with a port for attaching to the oxygen supply and can be used in adults and children. By using it upside-down it may be used to ventilate an infant (see Figure 14.4).

Self-inflating bags

Self-inflating bags come in several sizes (eg 240 ml, 500 ml, and 1600 ml). The size of the child determines the choice of bag. If the appropriate size is unavailable, a larger size may still be used in a small child by pinching the bag between a finger and thumb and carefully monitoring chest movement. A pressure-limiting valve set at 4 kPa (45 cmH$_2$O) is commonly provided as a protection against inadvertent barotrauma. It may (rarely) be overridden to ventilate lungs which have a high airway resistance or low compliance. The patient end of the bag connects to a one-way valve of a fish-mouth or leaf-flap design. The opposite end has a connection to the oxygen supply, and to a reservoir attachment. The reservoir enables high oxygen concentrations to be delivered. Without it, it is difficult to supply more than 50% oxygen to the patient, whatever the fresh gas flow, whereas with it an inspired oxygen concentration of 90% is easily achieved (see Chapter 14).

Other ventilation methods

A detailed discussion of mechanical ventilators is beyond the scope of this book. A simple, compact, robust, portable ventilator is a useful adjunct in the pre-hospital phase, provided its limitations are appreciated. They can give a false sense of security in the face of inadequate or excessive ventilation. Continual re-evaluation is therefore mandatory.

A T-piece and open-ended bag is often used in the hospital environment in children below 20 kg in weight, particularly by anaesthetists. While it allows some positive end-expiratory pressure (PEEP) to be exerted, it requires a "knack" to use it effectively and is useless if the oxygen supply fails. For these reasons, self-inflating bags are generally preferred in pre-hospital care. It is also possible to attach a PEEP valve to most self-inflating bags to help maintain oxygenation by preventing airway closure, though PEEP is not routinely required in the field.

Intravenous cannulae

These are included as tension pneumothorax may severely limit ventilation. Their use is described in Chapter 16.

Gastric tubes

Children are prone to air swallowing and vomiting. Air may also be forced into the stomach during bag and mask ventilation. This may cause vomiting, vagal stimulation or diaphragmatic splinting. A gastric tube will decompress the stomach and significantly improve both breathing and general wellbeing. Withholding the procedure "to be kind to the child" may cause more distress than performing it.

PRACTICAL SKILLS

The following practical skills are described in detail in Chapter 14:

- Oropharyngeal airway insertion
    small child
    older child
- Nasopharyngeal airway insertion
- Orotracheal intubation
    infant/small child
    older child
- Ventilation without intubation
    mouth-to-mask ventilation
    bag-and-mask ventilation

The basic skills of head and neck positioning, chin lift and jaw thrust are discussed in Chapter 6.

PUTTING IT TOGETHER: MANAGEMENT OF AIRWAY AND BREATHING

In order to respond urgently and retain thoroughness, effective emergency management demands a systematic, prioritised approach. Care can be structured into the four following phases.

Primary assessment

This consists of a rapid "physiological" examination to identify immediately life threatening emergencies. It should be completed in less than a minute and is prioritised as ABCDE:

- **A**irway
- **B**reathing
- **C**irculation
- **D**isability (nervous system)
- **E**xposure

From the respiratory viewpoint, do the following:

- **Look**, **listen** and **feel** for airway obstruction, respiratory arrest, depression or distress.
- **Assess** the work of breathing.
- **Count** the respiratory rate.
- **Listen** for stridor and/or wheeze.
- **Auscultate** for breath sounds.
- **Assess** skin colour.

If a significant problem is identified, management should be started immediately. After appropriate interventions have been performed, primary assessment can be resumed or repeated.

Box 7.3 AIRWAY AND BREATHING MANAGEMENT

Begin primary assessment . . .

Assess the airway . . .

If evidence of blunt trauma
   then protect the cervical spine from the outset
If any evidence of obstruction and altered consciousness
   then optimise the head and neck positioning
   and administer oxygen
   and consider chin lift, jaw thrust, suction, foreign body removal
If obstruction persists
   then consider oro- or nasopharyngeal airway
If obstruction still persists
   then consider intubation
If intubation impossible or unsuccessful
   then consider cricothyroidotomy
If stridor but relatively alert
   then allow self-ventilation whenever possible
   and encourage oxygen but do not force to wear mask
   and do not force to lie down
   and do not inspect the airway
      (except as a definitive procedure under controlled conditions)
   and assemble expert team and equipment

Assess the breathing . . .

If respiratory arrest or depression
   then administer oxygen by bag-valve-mask
   and consider intubation
If sedative or paralysing drugs possible
   then administer reversal agent
If respiratory distress or tachypnoea
   then administer oxygen
If lateralised ventilatory deficit
   then consider haemopneumothorax and inhaled foreign body
   and consider lung consolidation, collapse or pleural effusion
If chest injury
   then consider tension pneumothorax and massive haemothorax
   and consider flail segment and open pneumothorax
If evidence of tension pneumothorax
   then perform immediate needle decompression
If evidence of massive haemothorax
   then transfer rapidly, alerting hospital
If wheeze or crackles
   then consider asthma, bronchiolitis, pneumonia and heart failure
   but remember inhaled foreign body as a possible cause
If evidence of acute severe asthma
   then consider inhaled or intravenous beta-agonists
   and consider intravenous steroids
If evidence of heart failure
   then consider frusemide

Continue the primary assessment . . .

. . . proceed to assess the circulation and nervous system

If deteriorating from whatever cause
   then reassess the airway and breathing
   and be prepared to intubate and ventilate

Resuscitation

During this phase, life saving interventions are performed. These include such procedures as intubation, ventilation, cannulation, and fluid resuscitation. At the same time, oxygen is provided, vital signs are recorded, essential monitoring is established, and transfer to hospital is initiated.

From the respiratory viewpoint, do the following:

- Consider jaw- and neck-positioning manoeuvres.
- Administer oxygen.
- Consider suction and foreign body removal.
- Consider mask ventilation, and pharyngeal or tracheal intubation.
- Consider chest decompression.
- Consider needle cricothyroidotomy, if unable to oxygenate by alternative means. Initiate pulse oximetry and other monitoring at this time.

Secondary assessment

This consists of a thorough physical examination, together with appropriate investigations and will often not be undertaken before arrival in hospital. Conventionally, examination is from head to toe, and represents an "anatomical" assessment. Before embarking on this phase, it is important that the resuscitative measures are fully under way.

From the respiratory viewpoint, do the following:

- Perform a detailed examination of the airway, neck, and chest.
- Identify any swelling, bruising, or wounds.
- Re-examine for symmetry of breath sounds and movement.
- Do not forget to inspect and listen to the back of the chest.

Emergency treatment

All other urgent interventions are included in this phase.

If at any time the patient deteriorates, care returns to the primary assessment, and recycles through the system.

In the very sick or critically injured child, the primary assessment and management phases become integrally bound together. As a problem is identified, care shifts to the relevant intervention, before returning to the next part of the primary assessment. The simplified airway and breathing management protocol in Box 7.3 illustrates how this integration can be achieved. Careful documentation should be undertaken at all stages.

SUMMARY

- Correct selection and sizing of airway and ventilation equipment is essential.
- Management of airway and breathing has priority in the resuscitation of all patients.
- A systematic approach is required in the assessment and treatment of the airway and breathing.

Questions

1 What is the formula used to describe:

(a) The internal diameter of an endotracheal tube?
(b) The length of an endotracheal tube at the lips?

2 What size laryngeal mask airway is appropriate for a 4-year-old child?
3 Why should a self-inflating bag always have a reservoir bag attached to it during resuscitation?

8

The management of cardiac arrest

OBJECTIVES

After reading this chapter you should be able to:

- Identify the cardiac arrest rhythms
- Calculate the correct doses of adrenaline used in paediatric cardiac arrest
- Calculate the correct energy levels for defibrillation in paediatric cardiac arrest
- Describe the sequence of advanced life support treatments in paediatric cardiac arrest

INTRODUCTION

Cardiac arrest has occurred when there are no palpable central pulses. Before any specific therapy is started effective basic life support must be established as described in Chapter 6. Three cardiac arrest rhythms will be discussed in this chapter:

1 Asystole
2 Ventricular fibrillation
3 Electromechanical dissociation

PRE-HOSPITAL CONSIDERATIONS

Cardiac arrest in a child has a dismal prognosis. Every effort should therefore be made to prevent it occurring by early recognition of potentially serious illness and appropriate management. Occasionally it is, however, inevitable. It is particularly difficult to manage in the pre-hospital setting because ideally a team of skilled, well equipped people are required to provide optimum simultaneous management of the airway, breathing, circulation (cardiac massage), and drug administration. This abundance of resources is seldom, if ever, available outside hospital and therefore the recommended guidelines and protocols may not be possible to implement in full.

It must be remembered that, at the present time, the only factor known to improve the outcome of paediatric arrest is the time from the arrest to the arrival at hospital. This is regardless of the skill of the personnel or interventions performed. Thus the single most important "treatment", likely to improve the child's chances of survival is

not to delay in transferring the child to hospital. It is possible that if this is done, then other appropriate procedures may also help the child's outcome.

So when to move? This will depend on a number of issues, ranging from the size of the child to equipment available. Points to bear in mind are:

- If the child is small enough, remember, if possible, to "scoop and run" into the ambulance, rather than wasting time bringing equipment to the scene.
- As in all resuscitation, airway and breathing come before circulation and drugs.
- Good basic life support is essential and should not be sacrificed at the expense of performing advanced interventions such as intraosseous cannulation and adrenaline administration. However, some advanced interventions may improve the quality of the basic life support, such as endotracheal intubation if the child is to be transported a considerable distance. In this case the delay in transportation must be weighed against the benefit—in this particular scenario, the benefit would be a more secure airway (prevention of aspiration etc).
- If the child is in ventricular fibrillation, the most urgent treatment is defibrillation, and this should not be delayed for any reason. As for an adult, the sooner the child is defibrillated, the more likely the return to a rhythm with an output.
- It may be appropriate to perform one cycle of basic life support before moving the child—particularly if the arrest is thought to be due to hypoxia, as oxygenation is crucial.

The remainder of this chapter deals with what is considered to be the optimum management of asystole, ventricular fibrillation, and electromechanical dissociation with full facilities available. It is, however, important to appreciate that it will not always be possible to perform all the suggested interventions and drug regimes outside hospital without compromising transportation times and good basic life support with oxygen will remain the mainstay of management in the pre-hospital setting.

ASYSTOLE

This is the most common arrest rhythm in children, because the response of the young heart to prolonged severe hypoxia and acidosis is progressive bradycardia leading to asystole.

The ECG will distinguish asystole from ventricular fibrillation and electromechanical dissociation (Figure 8.1). The ECG appearance of ventricular asystole is an almost straight line; occasionally P waves are seen. Check that the appearance is not caused by an artefact, eg a loose wire or disconnected electrode. Turn up the gain on the ECG monitor.

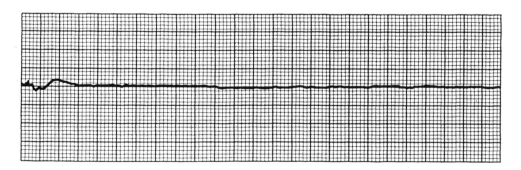

Figure 8.1. Asystole

Drugs in asystole

Before the administration of any drug, the patient must be receiving continuous and effective basic life support.

The protocol for drug use in asystole is shown in Figure 8.2.

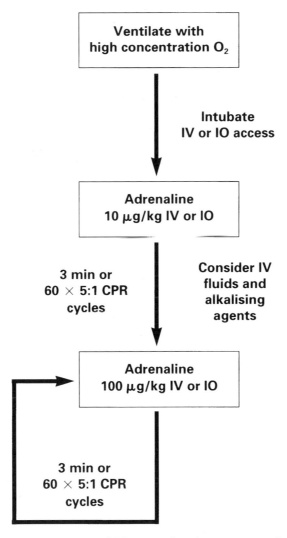

Figure 8.2. Protocol for drugs in asystole. CPR = cardiopulmonary resuscitation; IO = intraosseous; IV = intravenous

Adrenaline

Adrenaline is the first line drug for asystole. The initial intravenous dose is 10 mcg/kg (0.1 ml/kg of 1:10 000 solution). This is given through a peripheral or intraosseous line followed by a normal saline flush (2–5 ml). If there is no vascular access, the endotracheal tube can be used. Ten times the intravenous dose (ie 100 mcg/kg) should be given via this route. The drug should be injected quickly down a narrow-bore suction catheter beyond the tracheal end of the endotracheal tube and then flushed in with 1 or 2 ml of normal saline. In patients with pulmonary disease or prolonged asystole, pulmonary oedema and intrapulmonary shunting may make the endotracheal route less effective. If there has been no clinical effect, further doses should be given intravenously as soon as venous access has been secured.

53

Alkalising agents

Children with asystole may be profoundly acidotic as their cardiac arrest has usually been preceded by respiratory arrest or shock. However, the routine use of alkalising agents has not been shown to be of benefit. These agents should be administered only in cases where profound acidosis is likely, and should be considered if spontaneous circulation has not returned after the first dose of adrenaline. In the arrested patient arterial pH does not correlate well with tissue pH. Mixed venous or central venous pH should be used to guide any further alkalising therapy, and therefore is normally inappropriate for pre-hospital care. It should be remembered that good basic life support is more effective than alkalising agents at raising myocardial pH.

Bicarbonate is the most common alkalising agent currently available, the dose being 1 mmol/kg (2 ml/kg of a 4.2% solution). The tracheal route must not be used, and interactions with other drugs must be borne in mind.

INTERACTIONS AND LIMITATIONS OF BICARBONATE

- Bicarbonate must not be given in the same intravenous line as calcium because precipitation will occur
- Sodium bicarbonate inactivates adrenaline and dopamine, and therefore the line must be flushed with saline if these drugs are subsequently given
- Bicarbonate may not be given by the intratracheal route

Intravenous fluids

In some situations, where the cardiac arrest has resulted from circulatory failure, a standard (20 ml/kg) bolus of fluid should be given if there is no response to the initial dose of adrenaline. The nature of the fluid is less important than the volume, and either a crystalloid such as normal (0.9%) saline, or a colloid such as Gelofusin, can be given.

Second adrenaline dose

A second bolus of adrenaline (at a dose of ten times the first) should be given if spontaneous cardiac output has not returned 3 minutes after the first bolus. Ventilation and chest compressions must continue without interruption.

If there is still no response, continue to administer adrenaline 100 mcg/kg every 3 minutes ($60 \times 5{:}1$ CPR cycles). Evidence suggests that the outcome of asystole in childhood is very poor if there is no response to the second dose of adrenaline. Check that the intravenous line is still patent.

Calcium

There is no evidence that calcium is helpful in asystole. In fact, calcium can be detrimental, causing coronary artery spasm, and should only be used to treat documented hypocalcaemia, hyperkalaemia, or hypermagnesaemia. There is almost no indication for calcium in pre-hospital care.

Atropine

This drug is no longer in the asystole protocol. It can, however, be considered as an additional drug where there is evidence that increased vagal tone has been influential in the genesis of asystole, for example during airway manipulation. Its use must not detract from the application of measures of known efficacy.

The minimum dose to avoid a paradoxical parasympathetic action is 0.1 mg. The initial dose is 0.02 mg/kg and the maximum is 1 mg in children and 2 mg in adolescents.

VENTRICULAR FIBRILLATION

The ECG for ventricular fibrillation is shown in Figure 8.3.

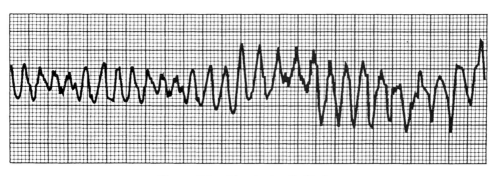

Figure 8.3. Ventricular fibrillation

This arrhythmia is uncommon in children but should be sought in those who are electrocuted, those who are recovering from hypothermia, those poisoned by tricyclic antidepressants, and those with cardiac disease. The protocol for ventricular fibrillation is shown in Figure 8.4.

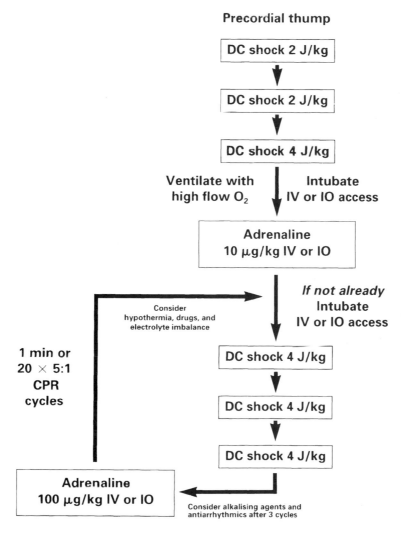

Figure 8.4. Protocol for ventricular fibrillation

Asynchronous electrical defibrillation should be carried out immediately. A precordial thump may be given in children if the onset of the arrhythmia is witnessed. Paediatric paddles (4.5 cm) should be used for children under 10 kg. One electrode is placed over the apex in the mid-axillary line, while the other is put immediately below the clavicle just to the right of the sternum. If only adult paddles are available for an infant under 10 kg, one may be placed on the infant's back and one over the left lower part of the chest at the front. See Part V, page 141.

The first two shocks should be given at 2 J/kg. If these two attempts are unsuccessful the third attempt should be at 4 J/kg. If three shocks fail to produce defibrillation, attention must turn to supporting coronary and cerebral perfusion, as in asystole. Basic life support should be continued. The airway should be secured and the patient ventilated with high flow oxygen. Adrenaline is given either as 10 mcg/kg intravenously or intraosseously or 100 mcg/kg via the tracheal route, then three further shocks (4 J/kg) are administered. If ventricular fibrillation still persists, then a higher dose of adrenaline (100 mcg/kg intravenously or intraosseously) should be given while 20 cardiopulmonary resuscitation cycles are carried out to maintain some coronary and cerebral perfusion. Once these are completed, a further three shocks (4 J/kg) should be administered. This is usually the point at which the child should be transported. The cycle of high dose adrenaline, cardiopulmonary resuscitation, and three defibrillatory shocks should be repeated until either ventricular fibrillation converts or resuscitation is discontinued.

During the resuscitation, the underlying cause of the arrhythmia should be considered. If VF is due to hypothermia then defibrillation may be resistant until core temperature is increased. Active rewarming should be commenced. If VF has been caused by drug overdose, then specific antiarrhythmic agents may be needed, so urgent transfer to hospital is required.

If there is resistance to defibrillation but no obvious reason for this, then different paddle positions or another defibrillator may be tried. There is some evidence that in infants large paddles may have an advantage because the larger contact area lowers transthoracic impedance resulting in a higher current flow for the same energy dose.

ELECTROMECHANICAL DISSOCIATION

This is the absence of a palpable pulse despite the presence of recognisable complexes on the ECG monitor. The most common cause in childhood is profound shock, which makes the pulse difficult to feel. Electromechanical dissociation (EMD) should be treated with rapid volume expansion (20 ml/kg of crystalloid or colloid) and adrenaline (10 mcg/kg) after basic life support, intubation and ventilation have been established. If there is no return of a palpable pulse, the next adrenaline dose should be 100 mcg/ kg.

Throughout management, the underlying cause should be sought. As mentioned above, hypovolaemia is the commonest cause in childhood. However, tension pneumothorax and cardiac tamponade should also be considered in the trauma patient. Rarely, pulmonary embolus may be the cause. In other patients electrolyte disturbance may be present. All of these need emergency care in a hospital, so the child should be moved urgently. During the journey, persistent EMD should be treated as in the protocol given in Figure 8.5.

POST-RESUSCITATION MANAGEMENT

Once spontaneous cardiac output has returned, frequent clinical reassessment must be carried out to detect deterioration or improvement until arrival at hospital. All patients should have continuing assessment of:

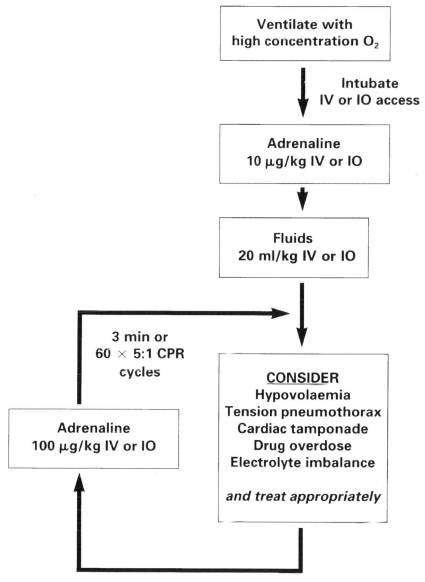

Figure 8.5. Protocol for electromechanical dissociation

- Pulse rate and rhythm—ECG monitor
- Oxygen saturation—pulse oximeter if available.

Often children who have been resuscitated from cardiac arrest die hours or days later from multiple organ failure. In addition to the cellular and homeostatic abnormalities that occur during the preceding illness, and during the arrest itself, cellular damage continues after spontaneous circulation has been restored. This is called reperfusion injury and is caused by the following:

- Depletion of ATP
- Entry of calcium into cells
- Free fatty acid metabolism activation
- Free oxygen radical production.

Post-resuscitation management aims to achieve and maintain homeostasis in order to optimise the chances of recovery. Management is directed in a systematic way in the emergency room and the intensive care unit.

WHEN TO STOP RESUSCITATION

If there have been no detectable signs of cardiac output, and there has been no evidence of cerebral activity despite up to 30 minutes of cardiopulmonary resuscitation, it is reasonable to stop resuscitation, and a suitably qualified doctor may elect to do so. Exceptions to this rule include the hypothermic child (in whom resuscitation must continue until the core temperature is at least 32 °C or cannot be raised despite active measures) and children who have taken overdoses of drugs. In these cases prolonged resuscitation attempts will be necessary and should always be continued for the full journey time to hospital.

The decision to stop resuscitation, in reality, is usually taken after the child has arrived in hospital.

SUMMARY

- Effective basic life support must be maintained at all times.
- The only factor known to improve the outcome of a paediatric out-of-hospital arrest is the length of time before hospital arrival.
- Asystole is the commonest arrest rhythm.
- Adrenaline is given at an initial dose of 10 mcg/kg then subsequent doses at 100 mcg/kg.
- Defibrillation doses are 2 J/kg for the first two shocks, then 4 J/kg.

Questions

1 What is the commonest cardiac arrest rhythm in children?
2 What doses of adrenaline are used in paediatric cardiac arrest?
3 How many J/kg are used in children to treat ventricular fibrillation?

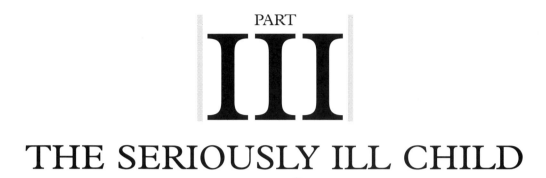

PART III

THE SERIOUSLY ILL CHILD

9

Recognition of the seriously ill child

OBJECTIVES

After reading this chapter you should be able to:

- State the normal respiratory and pulse rates for an infant, young child, and older child
- Identify the signs of respiratory, circulatory, and neurological failure in a child
- Recognise the significance of a fixed dilated pupil in a head injured child

As described in Chapters 1 and 8, the outcome for children suffering cardiac arrest is, in general, very poor. Earlier recognition and management of potential respiratory, circulatory, or central neurological failure will reduce mortality and secondary morbidity. This chapter describes the physical signs that should be used for rapid assessment of children.

RECOGNITION OF POTENTIAL RESPIRATORY FAILURE

Work of breathing

The degree of increase in the work of breathing allows clinical assessment of the severity of respiratory disease. The following should be assessed.

Respiratory rate

Tachypnoea at rest indicates that increased ventilation is needed either because of lung or airway disease, or because of metabolic acidosis. Normal respiratory rates at differing ages are shown in Table 9.1.

Table 9.1. Respiratory rate by age at rest

Age (years)	Respiratory rate (breaths per minute)
<1	30–40
2–5	25–30
5–12	20–25
>12	15–20

Recession

Intercostal, subcostal or sternal recession shows increased work of breathing. This sign is more easily seen in younger infants as they have a more compliant chest wall. Its presence in older children (ie over 6 or 7 years) suggests severe respiratory problems. The degree of recession gives some indication of the severity of respiratory difficulty.

Inspiratory or expiratory noises

An inspiratory noise while breathing (stridor) is a sign of laryngeal or tracheal obstruction. In severe obstruction the stridor may occur also in expiration, but the inspiratory component is usually more pronounced. Wheezing indicates lower airways narrowing and is more pronounced in expiration. A prolonged expiratory phase also indicates lower airways narrowing. The volume of the noise is not an indicator of severity.

Grunting

Grunting is produced by exhalation against a partially closed glottis. It is an attempt to generate a positive end-expiratory pressure and prevent airways' collapse at the end of expiration in children with "stiff" lungs. This is a sign of severe respiratory distress and is characteristically seen in infants.

Accessory muscle use

As in adult life, the sternomastoid muscles of the neck may be used as accessory respiratory muscles when the work of breathing is increased. In infants this may cause the head to bob up and down with each breath, making it ineffectual.

Flare of the alae nasi

Flaring of the alae nasi (nostrils) is seen especially in infants with respiratory distress.

Exceptions

There may be absent or decreased evidence of increased work of breathing in three circumstances:

● In the infant or child who has had severe respiratory problems for some time, fatigue may occur and the signs of increased work of breathing will decrease. **Exhaustion is a pre-terminal sign.**
● Children with **cerebral depression** from raised intracranial pressure, poisoning or encephalopathy will have respiratory inadequacy without increased work of breathing. The respiratory inadequacy in this case is caused by decreased respiratory drive.
● Children who have **neuromuscular disease** leading to weak respiratory muscles may present in respiratory failure without increased work of breathing.

The diagnosis of respiratory failure in such children is made by observing the effectiveness of breathing, and looking for other signs of respiratory inadequacy. These are discussed in the text.

Effectiveness of breathing

Auscultation of the chest will give an indication of the amount of air being inspired and expired. **A silent chest is an extremely worrying sign.** Similarly, observations of the degree of **chest expansion** (or in infants, abdominal excursion) add useful information.

Pulse oximetry can be used to measure the arterial oxygen saturation. The instruments are less accurate when SaO_2 is less than 70%, and in the presence of carboxyhaemoglobin. They also function poorly when there is poor peripheral circulation due to cold or shock.

Effects of respiratory inadequacy on other organs

Heart rate

Hypoxia produces tachycardia in the older infant and child. Anxiety and a fever will also contribute to tachycardia, making this a non-specific sign. Severe or prolonged hypoxia leads to bradycardia. **This is a pre-terminal sign**.

Skin colour

Hypoxia produces vasoconstriction and skin pallor. **Cyanosis is a late and pre-terminal sign of hypoxia**. By the time central cyanosis is visible in acute respiratory disease the patient is close to respiratory arrest. In the anaemic child cyanosis may never be visible, despite profound hypoxia. A few children will be cyanosed because of cyanotic heart disease. Their cyanosis will be largely unchanged by oxygen therapy, and may be obvious even when they are well.

Mental status

The hypoxic or hypercapnoeic child will be agitated and/or drowsy. Gradually drowsiness increases and eventually consciousness is lost. These extremely useful and important signs are often more difficult to detect in small infants. The parents may say that the infant is just "not himself". The examiner must assess the child's state of alertness by gaining eye contact and noting the response to voice and, if necessary, to painful stimuli. A generalised muscular hypotonia also accompanies hypoxic cerebral depression.

Reassessment

Single observations are useful, but much more information can be gained by frequent repeated observations to detect a trend in the patient's condition.

RECOGNITION OF POTENTIAL CIRCULATORY FAILURE (SHOCK)

Cardiovascular status

Heart rate

The heart rate initially increases in shock due to catecholamine release and as compensation for decreased stroke volume. The rate, particularly in small infants, may be extremely high (up to 220 beats per minute). Normal rates are shown in Table 9.2.

Table 9.2. Heart rate by age

Age (years)	Heart rate (beats per minute)
<1	110–160
2–5	95–140
5–12	80–120
>12	60–100

Eventually the heart may become so hypoxic and acidotic that it may slow. **Bradycardia is a preterminal sign**, usually heralding an asystolic cardiac arrest.

Pulse volume

Although blood pressure is maintained until shock is very severe, an indication of perfusion can be gained by comparative palpation of both peripheral and central pulses. Absent peripheral pulses and weak central pulses are serious signs of advanced shock, and indicate that hypotension is already present.

63

Capillary refill

Following cutaneous pressure on the forehead or chest, for 5 seconds, capillary refill should occur within 2 seconds. A slower refill time than this indicates poor skin perfusion. This is a particularly useful sign in septic shock. The interpretation of this sign must be made in the light of the ambient temperature—sick and traumatised children cool very quickly and this sign thus has limited use in the pre-hospital environment. The forehead and chest will be less affected than a digit by the temperature, and the use of the sign has been validated in these areas.

Blood pressure

Hypotension is a late and pre-terminal sign of circulatory failure. Once a child's blood pressure has fallen, cardiac arrest is imminent. Expected systolic blood pressure can be estimated by the formula:

$$\text{blood pressure} = 80 + (\text{age in years} \times 2)$$

Normal systolic pressures are shown in Table 9.3.

Table 9.3. Systolic blood pressure by age

Age (years)	Systolic blood pressure (mmHg)
<1	70–90
2–5	80–100
5–12	90–110
>12	100–120

Blood pressure measurement in children in the pre-hospital setting is of limited use. The correct cuff size must be used (the biggest that will fit comfortably on the upper arm of the child), the normal systolic pressure for the age of the child must be known (diastolic is not so easy and thus not so accurate in children), and the child must not be agitated. Finally, it is often difficult to palpate even a non-hypotensive child's pulse in a moving ambulance. To achieve all these criteria often takes more time than is appropriate outside hospital and a large range of blood pressure cuffs have to be carried. If the child is sufficiently shocked to be hypotensive, they will have other obvious signs of circulatory failure such as a raised pulse rate and prolonged capillary refill time which will be considerably more easy to monitor and provide much more sensitive indices of circulatory failure.

Effects of circulatory inadequacy on other organs

Respiratory system

A rapid respiration rate without recession is caused by the metabolic acidosis resulting from circulatory failure.

Skin

Mottled, cold, pale skin peripherally indicates poor perfusion. A line of coldness may be felt to move centrally as circulatory failure progresses.

Mental status

Agitation and then drowsiness leading to unconsciousness are characteristic of circulatory failure. These signs are caused by poor cerebral perfusion.

RECOGNITION OF POTENTIAL CENTRAL NEUROLOGICAL FAILURE

Neurological assessment should only be performed after airway (A), breathing (B), and circulation (C) have been assessed and treated. There are no neurological problems that take priority over ABC.

Both respiratory and circulatory failure will have central neurological effects. Conversely, some conditions with direct central neurological effects, such as meningitis, raised intracranial pressure (ICP) from trauma, and status epilepticus, may also have respiratory and circulatory consequences.

Neurological function

Conscious level

A rapid assessment of conscious level can be made by assigning the patient to one of the following categories:

A ALERT
V responds to VOICE
P responds to PAIN
U UNRESPONSIVE

The painful stimulus should be delivered either by pinching a digit or by pulling frontal hair. It may also be noted as an intravenous cannula is being placed. A child who is unresponsive or who only responds to pain has a significant degree of coma, equivalent to 8 or less on the Glasgow Coma Scale.

Posture

Many children who are suffering from a serious illness in any system are hypotonic (floppy). Stiffness and arching of the neck and back are signs of meningeal irritation, seen in conditions such as meningitis. Infants under the age of one do not always display this sign even in the presence of severe meningeal pathology. Stiff posturing such as that shown by decorticate (flexed arms, extended legs) or decerebrate (extended arms, extended legs) children is a sign of serious brain dysfunction. A painful stimulus may be necessary to elicit the posturing sign.

Pupils

Many drugs and cerebral lesions have effects on pupil size and reactions. However, the most important pupillary signs to seek are dilatation, unreactivity, and inequality, which indicate possible serious brain disorders.

It is particularly important that if, before the child reaches hospital, a pupil becomes fixed and dilated, the side on which this happens is noted. This sign indicates compression of the third nerve and occurs with compression of the upper part of the brain through the tentorial opening (uncal herniation) (Figure 9.1). The dilatation nearly always occurs on the same side as the damage. The hospital staff need to know which side developed a dilated pupil first, because if emergency treatment is required, it will help to guide them as to the side of the lesion.

Respiratory effects of central neurological failure

There are several recognisable breathing pattern abnormalities with raised ICP. However, they are often changeable and may vary from hyperventilation to Cheyne–Stokes (periodic) breathing to apnoea.

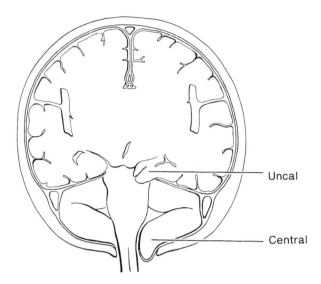

Figure 9.1. Herniation of the brain

Circulatory effects of central neurological failure

Systemic hypertension with sinus bradycardia (Cushing's response) indicates compression of the medulla oblongata caused by herniation of the cerebellar tonsils through the foramen magnum (central herniation) (Figure 9.1). **This is a late and pre-terminal sign**.

SUMMARY

The rapid clinical assessment of an infant or child

Airway and **B**reathing	Work of breathing
	Respiratory rate/rhythm
	Stridor/wheeze
	Auscultation
	Skin colour
Circulation	Heart rate
	Pulse volume
	Capillary refill
	Skin temperature
Disability	Mental status/conscious level
	Posture
	Pupils

The whole assessment should take less than a minute

Life threatening procedures and interventions must be initiated immediately, but once these have been undertaken the child can be transported to hospital. Generally the airway (A) and breathing (B) have to be stabilised before transportation whereas management of circulation (C) can often be done in transit, as can assessment of disability (D). Frequent reassessment of ABCD is necessary to assess progress and detect deterioration.

Questions

1 What is the normal respiratory rate for a 4-year-old child?
2 Where is the best place to test the capillary refill in a sick or injured child?
3 A head injured child develops a fixed dilated pupil on the right side. Which side of the brain is the injury likely to be?

10

The structured approach to the seriously ill child

OBJECTIVES

After reading this chapter you should be able to:

1 List the specific pre-hospital factors that pre-hospital personnel must take into account when deciding what treatment to provide before hospital
2 Name the five components to the structured approach to a seriously ill child
3 Describe the difference between the primary assessment and resuscitation and secondary assessment and emergency treatment
4 List the physical symptoms and signs which must be looked for in assessing the seriously ill child as part of the secondary assessment
5 Describe the treatments which may be required in (a) the primary assessment and (b) the secondary assessment

---

PRE-HOSPITAL CONSIDERATIONS

The treatment of children in the pre-hospital setting is challenging. Considerable flexibility in the application of knowledge and skills may be required because of the huge variety of circumstances and environments that may be encountered. In hospital, the environment, people available and equipment are, broadly speaking, similar from institution to institution. This is not always so in the pre-hospital environment. Although the approach to some medical problems may be identical in the two settings and be relatively inflexible, in other circumstances a great deal of common sense in interpretation of guidelines may be required. Many procedures cannot easily or safely be employed in the pre-hospital setting so children need rapid transportation to hospital and any intervention which will delay this must be justifiable.

There are a number of factors which the pre-hospital carer will have to take into account when considering the management—be it serious illness or trauma—which may not be relevant in hospital.

1 *The need for definitive care* Definitive care cannot be achieved in the pre-hospital setting. The aim of the pre-hospital carer is to ensure the child arrives in hospital as rapidly as possible, certainly without allowing the child to come to further harm and preferably by stabilising or even improving the condition en route.
2 *The environment* The safety of the rescuer is of prime importance and is a first consideration when approaching the patient. Secondly, the safety of the patient's

environment and those around must be secured and this may also delay or alter the child's management. Children make emotive patients and adults who are usually mindful of safety may take unnecessary risks when a child's life is perceived to be in danger. Is the environment compromising the child's state? For example, is the patient cold or wet? Children have a proportionately large surface area and become hypothermic very quickly when ill or injured.

3 *The distance/time from the hospital* A great deal of flexibility in the interpretation of guidelines for illness management is required when considering the distance (time) from the hospital. A judgement has to be made for each intervention as to whether the delay caused in transporting the child to hospital is outweighed by the benefit of the procedure. For example, if a non-breathing child is only 2 minutes from the hospital, it may not be justified to spend 10 minutes trying to intubate the child provided adequate ventilation can be achieved via a bag-valve-mask system. If the same child were an hour and a half from the hospital, intubation might be considered appropriate because of the difficulty of maintaining excellent ventilation via a mask for such a long time and the prolonged time during which the child would remain at risk of aspiration.

Entrapment may also pose difficulties. The patient may not be far from the hospital but if it is going to take 2 hours to free the child to allow transportation, it may be necessary to provide more treatment than if the child could be immediately moved. Analgesia and fluid resuscitation normally provided in the resuscitation room may be required because of the delay and this should not be withheld if it is clinically indicated. It is, however, important not to unnecessarily delay the extrication of the patient by overzealous treatment.

4 *Equipment available* Equipment available in the pre-hospital setting is very limited compared to that available in hospital. Doctors tend to carry different quantities and types of equipment, as do ambulances in different ambulance services. Paediatric equipment may be even more limited than that available to adults.

5 *Skills of the pre-hospital personnel* The training and background of different personnel will vary as will the frequency and expertise with which they perform those skills.

6 *Other factors* Other unusual circumstances may have to be considered—for example, is this a multi-casualty incident? If many people require medical attention some form of triage will be necessary and restrictions on the priorities of care may have to be made because of logistics of transportation, personnel available, and equipment available etc.

> • The time that sick children spend prior to hospital should be minimised, but not by compromising their overall medical condition
> • Every intervention and treatment which slows the immediate transportation of the patient to definitive medical care must be judged against risks to the patient of delay

TREATMENT

The treatment of a child in an emergency requires a rapid assessment and urgent intervention. The structured approach includes:

1 Primary assessment.
2 Resuscitation.
3 Secondary assessment.
4 Emergency treatment.
5 Definitive care.

Primary assessment and resuscitation include management of vital ABC functions and assessment of disability (CNS function). This takes place before any diagnostic assessment or treatment is initiated. Once the patient's vital functions are stable, *secondary assessment and emergency treatment* begin. Immediately treatable illnesses are excluded or emergency treatment commenced. This will be while the child is still being transported to hospital. During the secondary assessment vital signs must be checked frequently to detect any change in the child's condition. If the child deteriorates, then a return to the primary survey and resuscitation should be made.

Definitive care is invariably undertaken in hospital and is beyond the scope of this book.

PRIMARY ASSESSMENT AND RESUSCITATION

In a severely ill child a rapid examination of vital functions is required. This is usually performed before moving the child. The physical signs described in Chapter 9 are used in an ABC approach. The primary assessment and resuscitation must be instituted before the more detailed secondary assessment is performed.

Airway

Primary assessment

Patency of the airway must be assessed. It is important to remember that the "Look, Listen, Feel" method of assessing airway patency is only effective if there is some spontaneous ventilation present.

- If the child can speak this indicates that the airway is patent, that breathing is occurring, and that there is adequate circulation. The child may not respond to a health professional but may be induced to speak by the accompanying adult.
- If the child is too young or frightened to give a response then he or she may cry: this is an equally adequate indication that the airway is patent.
- If there is no evidence of air movement, chin lift or jaw thrust manoeuvres should be carried out and the airway reassessed. If there continues to be no evidence of air movement, then airway patency can be assessed by performing an opening manoeuvre and giving rescue breaths (see Basic life support, Chapter 6).

Resuscitation

If the airway is not patent when assessed by the "Look, Listen, Feel" technique, but patency can be secured by a chin lift or jaw thrust, then an airway adjunct may be required to maintain it. Intubation should be considered if this fails and the child is a long distance from the hospital or patency cannot be secured by any other method.

Breathing

Primary assessment

A patent airway does not ensure adequate ventilation. The latter requires an intact respiratory centre and adequate pulmonary function augmented by coordinated movement of the diaphragm and chest wall. The adequacy of breathing can be assessed as shown in Box 10.1.

> **Box 10.1 ASSESSMENT OF THE ADEQUACY OF BREATHING**
>
> - **The work of breathing**
>   Recession
>   Respiratory rate
>   Inspiratory or expiratory noises
>   Grunting
>   Accessory muscle use
>   Flare of the alae nasi
>
> - **Effectiveness of breathing**
>   Breath sounds
>   Chest expansion
>   Abdominal excursion
>
> - **Effects of inadequate respiration**
>   Heart rate
>   Skin colour
>   Mental status

The normal range of respiratory rate by age is given in Table 10.1.

Table 10.1. Respiratory rate by age

Age (years)	Respiratory rate (breaths per minute)
<1	30–40
2–5	25–30
5–12	20–25
>12	15–20

A pulse oximeter should be attached, if available, and the oxygen saturation while breathing air noted. A saturation of less than 90% while breathing air or less than 95% while breathing oxygen is a worrying sign.

Resuscitation

High-flow oxygen should be given to all children with respiratory difficulty or hypoxia. In the non-intubated child this should be delivered via a non-rebreathing mask with a reservoir bag. Parents can be invaluable in assisting with the administration of oxygen in this setting.

In the child with inadequate respiratory effort, ventilation should be supported by bag-valve-mask oxygenation. Rarely intubation and intermittent positive pressure ventilation may be required. This is not usually feasible outside hospital because of the need for anaesthesia.

In the non-breathing patient logistics such as ease of maintaining the airway, vomiting, and the distance from the hospital will dictate the need for intubation.

Circulation

Primary assessment

Circulation is assessed as shown in Box 10.2.

Box 10.2 ASSESSMENT OF THE ADEQUACY OF CIRCULATION

- **Cardiovascular status**
  Heart rate
  Pulse volume
  Capillary refill
  (Blood pressure)

- **Effects of circulatory inadequacy on other organs**
  Respiratory system
  Skin
  Mental status
  Urinary output

The normal circulatory parameters are as shown in Table 10.2. The child's heart rate and pulse volume should be assessed by palpating both central and peripheral pulses. Capillary refill time (CRT) should be assessed, with due allowance for ambient temperature. Normal CRT is less than 2 seconds. It is most reliably done on the forehead or the sternum. An ECG monitor should be attached.

Table 10.2. Heart rate and systolic blood pressure by age

Age (years)	Heart rate (beats per minute)	Systolic blood pressure (mmHg)
<1	110–160	70–90
2–5	95–140	80–100
5–12	80–120	90–110
>12	60–100	100–120

The blood pressure should only be measured if it will not delay the child's transfer to hospital and logistics and equipment allow an accurate reading (see Chapter 9).

Resuscitation

Every child with an inadequate circulation (shock) should have high flow oxygen administered through a non-rebreathing mask with a reservoir bag (or via a bag-valve-mask or endotracheal tube if necessary).

Venous or intraosseous access should be gained if appropriate, usually in transit to hospital. The glucose level should be checked on insertion of the needle. Crystalloid or colloid (20 ml/kg) should be given, except in children with suspected cardiogenic shock (ie arrhythmias, history of heart disease; see Chapter 11, section on Shock). Document the volume administered.

Disability (neurological evaluation)

Primary assessment

Hypoxia, shock, and hypoglycaemia all cause a decrease in conscious level. Any problem with ABC must be addressed before assuming that a decrease in conscious level is due to a primary neurological problem.

The assessment proceeds as follows:

- The level of consciousness should be recorded using the AVPU scale:

  A ALERT
  V responds to VOICE
  P responds to PAIN
  U UNRESPONSIVE

- Pupillary size and reaction should be noted as a baseline.
- The presence and side of convulsive movements should be noted.
- Any patient with a decreased conscious level or convulsions, or having vascular access obtained must have an initial glucose stick test performed.

Resuscitation

Prolonged (>5–10 minutes) or recurrent fits require active intervention. Diazepam should be given rectally rather than intravenously in the first instance as it is less likely to depress ventilation. This should usually be done during transportation.

Hypoglycaemia should be treated with 0.5 g/kg of dextrose (i.e. 5 ml/kg of 10% dextrose).

SECONDARY ASSESSMENT AND EMERGENCY TREATMENT

The secondary assessment takes place once vital functions have been assessed and the initial treatment of life threatening emergencies has been started. It includes a more detailed medical history and a thorough clinical examination. Emergency treatments will be appropriate at this stage—either to treat specific conditions (such as wheezing) or processes (such as raised intracranial pressure). The establishment of a definite diagnosis is part of definitive care and usually will wait until hospital.

The history often provides vital clues which help the carer to identify the disease process in the patient and provide the appropriate emergency care. In the case of children, the history is often obtained from an accompanying parent, although a history should also be sought from the child if possible. Pre-hospital personnel should be prepared to provide "their own" history of the child's initial condition and any response to treatment on arrival at hospital.

Some children will present with an acute exacerbation of a known condition such as asthma or epilepsy. Such information is helpful in focusing attention on the appropriate system but the carer should be wary of dismissing new pathologies in such patients. The structured approach prevents this problem. Unlike trauma (which is dealt with later), illness affects systems rather than anatomical areas. The secondary assessment must reflect this and the history of the complaint should be sought with special attention to the presenting system or systems involved. After the presenting system has been dealt with, all other systems should be assessed, and if time allows any additional emergency treatments commenced as appropriate.

The secondary assessment is not intended to complete the diagnostic process, but rather is intended to identify any problems that require further emergency treatment.

The following gives an outline of a structured approach which can be used prior to hospital. It is not exhaustive but addresses the majority of emergency conditions which are amenable to specific emergency treatments in this time period.

The symptoms, signs and treatments relevant to each emergency condition are elaborated on in Chapter 11.

Respiratory (breathing)

Secondary assessment

Box 10.3 gives common symptoms and signs which should be sought in the respiratory system. Emergency investigations are also suggested below.

Box 10.3 SECONDARY ASSESSMENT: RESPIRATORY

Symptoms	Signs
Breathlessness	Apnoea
Coryza, cough	Cyanosis
Drooling, hoarseness	Stridor
Inability to drink	Flaring of nostrils, grunting
because of pain	Tachypnoea
Abdominal pain	Recession
Chest pain	Grunting
Feeding difficulties	Tracheal shift
	Chest wall crepitus
	Abnormal percussion note
	Wheeze
	(Crepitations on auscultation)
	Tachycardia, bradycardia
	Agitation, drowsiness

( ) may be difficult to elicit outside hospital

Investigations

Peak flow if asthma suspected, glucose stick (except with stridor)

Emergency treatment

- If "bubbly" noises are heard, the airway is full of secretions requiring clearance by suction.
- If there is a harsh stridor associated with a barking cough and severe respiratory distress, upper airway obstruction due to severe croup should be suspected. Rapid transportation is needed and the hospital should be alerted.
- If there is a quiet stridor in a sick-looking child, consider epiglottitis. Do not jeopardise the airway by unpleasant or frightening interventions. Again alert the hospital and transport the child urgently.
- With a sudden onset and significant history of inhalation, consider a laryngeal foreign body. If the choking child procedure has been unsuccessful, the patient may require laryngoscopy. Do not jeopardise the airway by unpleasant or frightening interventions but transport immediately and alert the hospital. However, in extreme cases of life threat with apnoea immediate direct laryngoscopy to remove a visible foreign body with Magill's forceps may be necessary.
- Stridor following ingestion/injection of a known allergen suggests anaphylaxis. Children in whom this is likely should receive IM adrenaline (10 mcg/kg).
- Children with a history of asthma or with wheeze and significant respiratory distress, depressed peak flow and/or hypoxia should receive nebulised beta$_2$-agonists such as salbutamol 2.5–5 mg driven with oxygen.

Cardiovascular (circulation)

Secondary assessment

Box 10.4 gives common symptoms and signs which should be sought in the cardiovascular system.

Box 10.4   SECONDARY ASSESSMENT: CARDIOVASCULAR

Symptoms	Signs
Breathlessness	Abnormal colour and perfusion
Sweatiness	Abnormal pulse volume and rhythm
Feeding difficulties	Tachycardia or bradycardia
Drowsiness	Peripheral oedema/dehydration
Floppiness	(Hypotension/hypertension)
Palpitations	(Raised jugular venous pressure)
Fluid loss	(Crepitations on auscultation)
	(Cardiac murmur)
	(Hepatomegaly)
	Abnormal respiratory rate and depth
	Altered conscious level/hypotonia

( ) may be difficult to elicit outside hospital

Emergency treatment

- Further boluses of fluid in a dose of 20 ml/kg should be given to shocked children who have not had a sustained improvement to the first bolus given at resuscitation and who are not thought to have a primary cardiac cause for their condition, ie no history of cardiac disease or rhythm disturbance.
- Consider IV penicillin given slowly (Table 10.3) in shocked children with no obvious fluid loss. Sepsis is likely. Have they got a purpuric rash suggestive of meningococcaemia?
- If anaphylaxis is suspected in the shocked patient adrenaline should be given intramuscularly in a dose 10 mcg/kg, in addition to fluid boluses intravenously.

Table 10.3.   Dose of penicillin for treatment of meningococcal disease

Age	IV/IO/IM route
<1 year	300 mg
1–9 years	600 mg
10 years or over	1.2 g

NB: Check that there is no history of penicillin allergy before giving

Neurological (disability)

Secondary assessment

Box 10.5 gives common signs and symptoms which should be sought in the nervous system.

Box 10.5   SECONDARY ASSESSMENT: NEUROLOGICAL

Symptoms	Signs
Headache	Altered conscious level
Change in behaviour	Convulsions
Drowsiness/loss of alertness	Altered pupil size and reactivity
Weakness	Posture
Visual disturbance	Oculo-cephalic reflexes*
Convulsions	Meningism (neck/back stiffness)
Altered conscious level	(Papilloedema or retinal haemorrhage)*
	Altered deep tendon reflexes*
	(Hypertension)

( ) may be difficult to elicit outside hospital
*Only if time

Emergency treatment
- If convulsions persist, repeat rectal diazepam 0.4 mg/kg.
- If there is evidence of raised intracranial pressure, that is, an unconscious child with a decreasing conscious level and abnormal posturing, then the patient should be transported without delay and the hospital alerted.
- In unconscious children with pin-point pupils, consider opiate poisoning. A trial of naloxone should be given.
- **Check the glucose in all children with a depressed conscious level.** If it is low give dextrose.

External (exposure)

Secondary assessment
The common signs of serious illness which should be sought externally are:

- Petechial or purpuric rash.
- Urticarial rash.
- Swelling of lips or tongue.
- Fever.

Emergency treatment
- In a child with circulatory and/or neurological symptoms and signs, a petechial or purpuric rash suggests meningococcal septicaemia. The patient should receive penicillin in the dose given in Table 10.3.
- In a child with respiratory or circulatory difficulty, the presence of an urticarial rash or angio-oedema suggests anaphylaxis. Give adrenaline (10 mcg/kg) IM, consider fluids and salbutamol, and follow the anaphylaxis protocol.

Gastrointestinal

Gastrointestinal emergencies usually present with shock from fluid loss or occasionally blood loss. This will become apparent during the primary assessment of the circulation or the secondary assessment of the cardiovascular system. The symptoms and signs shown in Box 10.6 may be useful.

Box 10.6   SECONDARY ASSESSMENT: GASTROINTESTINAL

Symptoms	Signs
Vomiting, particularly bile-stained	Abdominal tenderness
Blood PR	Abdominal mass
Abdominal pain	

Further history

Developmental and social history
Particularly in a small child or infant, knowledge of the child's developmental progress and immunisation status may be useful. The family circumstances may also be helpful, sometimes prompting parents to remember other details of the family's medical history.

Drugs and allergies
Any medication that the child is currently on or has been on should be recorded, and in addition any medication in the home that the child might have had access to if poisoning is a possibility.

SUMMARY

The structured approach to the seriously ill child outlined here allows the pre-hospital carer to focus on the appropriate level of diagnosis and treatment before the ill child arrives in hospital. Primary assessment and resuscitation are concerned with the maintenance of vital functions, while secondary assessment and emergency treatment allow more specific urgent therapies to be started. This latter phase of care requires a system-by-system approach to this and minimises the chances of significant conditions being missed

Questions

1   What is the difference between the primary assessment and the secondary assessment?
2   In what way may the distance (time) from the hospital influence the management of a seriously ill child?
3   Name six symptoms of circulatory failure in a child.

11

Treating seriously ill children

OBJECTIVES

After reading this chapter you should be able to:

- Describe the pre-hospital management of a child with (a) upper, (b) lower airway problems
- List the five types of shock and outline their treatments
- Describe how to manage (a) convulsions, (b) coma in a child
- List three treatments for hypoglycaemia
- Describe the management of a poisoned child

DIAGNOSIS

Diagnosis in the pre-hospital setting can conveniently be divided into three categories.

Most illnesses encountered in the emergency treatment of paediatric patients do not need diagnostic labels. Treating life threatening conditions and transportation are the first priorities. An example of this would be a child who is wheezing. The job of the pre-hospital carer is to provide prompt transportation to hospital and if possible provide treatment for the wheezing child without compromising the length of time it will take to reach the destination. It is the job of the hospital to identify why the child is wheezing so that a definitive management plan can be initiated and, if necessary, preventative measures against future attacks can be taken.

A second smaller group of illnesses *will require some understanding of their cause*, but not a complete diagnosis. An example of this would be a child who is fitting because of hypoglycaemia. It is important to diagnose the hypoglycaemia as early as possible in order to treat it and minimise the chances of brain damage. However, unless the low blood sugar is obviously due to some cause which requires equally urgent pre-hospital care, the hospital can sort out why the child became hypoglycaemic, provide ongoing management, and advise on measures to prevent a recurrence.

The final group of illnesses, which are very small in number, do actually require a definitive diagnosis or a *high index of suspicion* because the appropriate specific treatment for that condition is so urgent that the child's chances of survival might deteriorate significantly if the treatment is delayed until hospital admission, ie any loss of time in transportation is outweighed by the potential benefit. Examples are meningococcal septicaemia, for which penicillin is required, and anaphylactic shock, for which adrenaline is needed. Personnel who may have to deal with these illnesses should ensure that the necessary drugs for treating these conditions are available.

RESPIRATORY PROBLEMS

Respiratory emergencies account for 30–40% of acute medical admissions to hospital in children and over 450 children will die each year as a result of them, the majority being under 12 months old.

Reasons why children are prone to respiratory problems are:

- Children are susceptible to infections to which many adults have subsequently become immune.
- The upper and lower airways in children are smaller and are more easily obstructed by mucosal swelling, secretion or foreign bodies.
- The thoracic cage of young children is much more compliant than that of adults. When there is airways obstruction and an increase in respiratory effort, this increased compliance results in marked chest wall recession and a reduction in the efficiency of breathing.
- The respiratory muscles of young children are relatively inefficient. In infancy the diaphragm is the principal respiratory muscle and the intercostal and accessory muscles make relatively little contribution. Respiratory muscle fatigue can develop rapidly and results in respiratory failure and apnoea.

Causes of respiratory difficulty

Outside hospital, the causes can be divided into upper airway obstruction, such as croup, foreign body or epiglottitis (rare since the introduction of the Hib vaccination), and lower airway pathology, such as asthma, bronchiolitis or pneumonia.

Assessment

Assessment, as for all emergencies, follows ABC and D. The seriousness of the respiratory problem can be assessed using the techniques described in the chapters on Recognition of the Seriously Ill Child (Chapter 9) and the Structured Approach to the Seriously Ill Child (Chapter 10).

UPPER AIRWAY OBSTRUCTION

Causes

The causes of upper airway obstruction are listed in Table 11.1.

Table 11.1. Causes of upper airway obstruction

Incidence	Diagnosis
Very common	Croup (viral)
Common	Croup (recurrent or spasmodic)
Uncommon	Foreign body
Rare	Croup (bacterial)
	Inhalation of hot gases
	Angioneurotic oedema
	Trauma
	Epiglottitis
	Infectious mononucleosis
	Retropharyngeal abscess
	Diphtheria

Croup

This is the commonest cause of stridor and the term describes an illness which leads to an inspiratory stridor, barking cough, and variable respiratory distress. More than 95% of croup is due to a viral infection, but less commonly children may be prone to recurrent croup. Rarely the illness may be due to a bacterial infection—over 80% of these latter children will require intubation at some point, as opposed to about 5% of those with viral croup.

Treatment

The main aim of treatment of the child with stridor is to transport the child to hospital without worsening the condition or precipitating a respiratory arrest. Two major factors which may contribute to this and can be minimised or avoided are increased agitation of the child and inserting things into the child's mouth, eg spatulas etc. Examination should be kept to a minimum and confined to only that which the child will allow. The remainder of the examination of a child with stridor should be made by simple observation.

Treatment should also be geared towards these ends. The child should be kept calm and every effort made to avoid upsetting him or her. Crying will increase oxygen demand and may increase laryngeal swelling. The airway will be best maintained in the conscious child by the child himself who may prefer to sit in a certain position. This should be permitted. If the child wants to sit on the parent's knee, this is also appropriate. A favourite teddy bear or similar reassuring article should be brought with the child to hospital if desired. The parents are a mainstay of treatment—they are usually best at keeping their children calm and reassured—every encouragement should be made for them to participate in their child's care. Oxygen may be given via a face mask if tolerated and by wafting the mask near the face if not. If even this distresses the child, then common sense has to dictate its importance.

The use of nebulised budesonide and adrenaline in presumed viral croup in the pre-hospital setting remains controversial. Budesonide has been shown to lead to some clinical improvement within several hours which may be sustained for 24 hours. It is uncertain whether it will lead to a significant improvement prior to most hospital admissions, and nebulisers can distress some children. The potential benefit of the budesonide in the child's overall illness against the risk of upsetting him must be weighed up, and in some areas where the time to hospital admission is not great, it may be considered better to wait until the child has arrived safely in hospital. Nebulised adrenaline (5 ml of 1:1000) produces a transient improvement in severe croup for 30–60 minutes, but this rarely alters the long term course of the illness. It is often used in hospital to "buy time" while advanced airway treatment is being organised. Whilst it sounds superficially ideal for the pre-hospital emergency treatment of severe croup, it must be remembered that, again, the nebuliser may cause distress and, more importantly that adrenaline is arrhythmogenic and the hypoxic myocardium may tolerate it poorly; the drug may thus predispose to arrhythmias.

Even if the child appears to be deteriorating, it is important not to upset him or her further by frightening or painful interventions—for example, the child should not have a glucose stick performed or an IV cannula placed. These procedures are likely to cause distress and crying and could precipitate a respiratory arrest. If the child is thought to have inhaled a foreign body *and is able to breathe*, no attempt should be made to remove it prior to hospital in case it slides away and causes complete airway obstruction.

If the child *does* have a respiratory arrest it is often possible to use bag-and-mask ventilation to maintain adequate oxygenation, despite the fact that there is airway obstruction. If a foreign body is thought to be the cause of the obstruction it may be appropriate at this point to gently inspect the upper airway to see if the foreign body can be removed with Magill's forceps.

> **Do not attempt to intubate a child with stridor unless bag-and-mask ventilation has proved impossible**

Children with stridor may have a very difficult airway to intubate and will need a much smaller endotracheal tube than usual because of the obstruction. Even in very experienced hands, a child with epiglottitis (a bacterial infection that produces stridor) may be impossible to intubate.

Rapid transportation is essential and if the airway obstruction appears to be severe the hospital should be alerted so that they can have a suitably skilled team available to undertake advanced airway management on arrival.

LOWER AIRWAY OBSTRUCTION

This is likely to be due to asthma or infection (either bacterial or viral). An acute exacerbation of asthma is the most common reason for a child to be admitted to hospital in the UK and has increased seven-fold in younger children between 1970 and 1986. It now represents 10–20% of all acute medical admissions in children, and 40–50 children will die each year.

Management of lower respiratory tract symptoms is, as usual, by ABC. The airway should be maintained and 100% oxygen given via a non-rebreathing mask. Some compromise may be required if the child does not tolerate the mask. Again the parents may be helpful in encouraging the child to accept the oxygen, or they may help by holding up the mask near the child. The respiration rate, heart rate, and conscious level should be monitored continuously and saturation monitoring performed if available. If a wheeze is present, nebulised salbutamol 2.5–5 mg should be given using 4–6 l/min of oxygen in all but the mildest of cases. The nebuliser can be given during transfer and can be repeated if there is insufficient improvement and time allows. Nebulised salbutamol is not recommended for children less than 6 months of age as it is relatively ineffective in this age group. Ipratropium bromide may be considered in these circumstances. If the child is thought to have severe or life threatening respiratory problems, (Boxes 11.1 and 11.2) the hospital should be made aware of the child's condition.

Box 11.1 FEATURES OF SEVERE RESPIRATORY DIFFICULTY

- Unable to talk in sentences (age appropriate)
- Recession
- Respiratory rate >50 breaths per minute
- Heart rate >140 beats per minute

Box 11.2 FEATURES OF LIFE THREATENING RESPIRATORY DIFFICULTY

- Severe recession
- Depressed conscious level
- Marked use of accessory muscles
- Oxygen saturation <85% in air/cyanosis
- Silent chest
- Poor respiratory effort
- Depressed conscious level

OXYGEN SATURATION MONITORING

Pulse oximetry measures the oxygen saturation of arterial blood continuously and a measured saturation of 95% or more is strongly suggestive of adequate peripheral arterial oxygenation. There are various conditions which can interfere with pulse oximetry and it is important to check that the pulse rate on the pulse oximeter correlates with the patient's measured pulse. Particular pitfalls include severe hypothermia, carbon monoxide poisoning and profound anaemia, all of which may give erroneous readings.

SHOCK

> **Shock results from failure of circulatory function leading to inadequate amounts of nutrients, especially oxygen, being delivered to the tissues, with inadequate removal of tissue waste products**

There are three categories of shock in children.

Phase 1 (compensated shock)

In this phase sympathetic reflexes maintain the blood pressure and divert blood to essential organs, such as the brain and heart. The kidneys also conserve water and salt and intestinal fluid is reabsorbed from the digestive tract. The patient may be mildly agitated, pale, and tachycardic. The child will have a prolonged capillary refill time, but a normal systolic blood pressure with a normal or raised diastolic blood pressure.

Phase 2 (uncompensated shock)

In worsening shock, compensatory mechanisms are starting to fail and some areas of the body that normally have poor blood supply cannot metabolise properly. The patient in phase 2 shock has a falling blood pressure, very poor capillary return, tachycardia, cold peripheries, acidotic breathing, depressed conscious level, and a decreased or absent urine output. In a child, because of children's excellent ability to compensate for shock, **this is a pre-terminal stage** and must be managed very aggressively.

Phase 3 (irreversible shock)

The diagnosis of irreversible shock is a retrospective one because the damage to key organs such as the heart and brain is of such magnitude that death occurs despite adequate restoration of the circulation. The metabolic disturbance which has taken place prior to restoration of the circulation is so great that the body cannot recover.

> **Early recognition and effective management of shock are vital**

Causes of shock

Maintenance of adequate tissue perfusion depends on the pump (the heart) delivering the correct type and volume of fluid (blood) through controlled vessels (arteries, veins, and capillaries) without abnormal obstruction to flow. Inadequate tissue perfusion resulting in impaired cellular metabolism (ie shock) may result from defects of the pump (cardiogenic), loss of fluid (hypovolaemic), abnormalities of vessels (distributive), flow restriction (obstructive), or inadequate oxygen releasing capacity (dissociative).

From Table 11.2 it can be seen that the most common causes of shock in the paediatric patient are hypovolaemia from any cause (including trauma) and septicaemia (distributive).

Table 11.2. Classification of causes of shock (common causes are emboldened)

Hypovolaemic	**Haemorrhage**
	Diarrhoea
	Vomiting
	Burns
	Peritonitis
Distributive	**Septicaemia**
	Anaphylaxis
	Vasodilating drugs
	Anaesthesia
	Spinal cord injury
Cardiogenic	Arrhythmias
	Cardiomyopathy
	Heart failure
	Valvular disease
	Myocardial contusion
	Myocardial infarction (very rare)
Obstructive	**Tension pneumothorax**
	Haemopneumothorax
	Flail chest
	Cardiac tamponade
	Pulmonary embolus
	Hypertension
Dissociative	Profound anaemia
	Carbon monoxide poisoning
	Methaemoglobinaemia

History

The history is essential in treating the shocked patient. Knowledge of the child's previous illness and the history of the present illness or injury will give important clues as to the underlying cause of the shocked state. This is necessary in order to direct therapy appropriately.

Assessment

The airway, breathing, and circulation should be assessed as normal. An assessment of the degree of circulatory compromise can be made by checking the features outlined in Box 11.3.

Box 11.3 ASSESSMENT OF THE ADEQUACY OF CIRCULATION

- **Cardiovascular status**
  Heart rate
  Pulse volume
  Capillary refill
  (Blood pressure)
- **Effects of circulatory inadequacy on other organs**
  Respiratory rate and character
  Skin appearance and temperature
  Mental status

Normal values of vital signs

The normal values for vital signs are summarised in Table 11.3. All single parameters should be interpreted within the whole clinical context.

Table 11.3. Vital signs: approximate range of normal

Age (years)	Respiratory rate (breaths/min)	Systolic BP (mmHg)	Pulse (/min)
<1	30–40	70–90	110–160
2–5	25–30	80–100	95–140
5–12	20–25	90–110	80–120
>12	15–20	100–120	60–100

Weight and blood volume

These can be calculated using the following formulae:

$$\text{Weight in kg} = 2\,(\text{age in years} + 4)$$
$$\text{Blood volume (ml)} = 80 \times \text{weight in kg}$$

Clinical signs of hypovolaemic shock

Data on the stages of shock in infants and children are limited, but the clinical signs shown in Table 11.4 are useful in the assessment of hypovolaemic shock.

Table 11.4. Signs of shock from blood loss

Clinical sign	Compensated	Uncompensated	Pre-terminal (?irreversible)
Blood loss(%)	Up to 25	25–40	>40
Heart rate	Tachycardia +	Tachycardia + +	Tachycardia/bradycardia
Systolic BP	Normal	Normal or falling	Plummeting
Pulse volume	Normal/reduced	Reduced +	Reduced + +
Capillary refill time	Normal/increased	Increased +	Increased + +
Skin	Cool, pale	Cold, mottled	Cold, deathly pale
Respiratory rate	Tachypnoea +	Tachypnoea + +	Sighing respiration
Mental state	Mild agitation	Lethargic Uncooperative	Reacts only to pain or unresponsive

Heart rate

Tachycardia is a common response to many types of stress. In shock it is a compensatory mechanism to attempt to maintain an adequate stroke volume.

Bradycardia is a pre-terminal sign

Peripheral pulses

Diminished peripheral pulses are a good indicator of shock. Because of the variability of blood pressure with age in children, the presence of a particular pulse cannot be used to predict the minimum value of the systolic blood pressure (as is sometimes done in adults). Peripheral pulses may sometimes be bounding in early septic shock because of a hyper-dynamic circulation.

Skin perfusion and capillary refill

A capillary refill of more than 2 seconds is evidence of reduced skin perfusion. Capillary refill should be done on the forehead or chest. Its use is limited in cold environments, but otherwise it can be a valuable tool, particularly when reassessing the response to treatment. Mottled, pale and bluish skin are all signs of poor skin perfusion and are useful signs provided the environment is warm.

Blood pressure

The value of blood pressure measurement is limited in the pre-hospital setting: see Chapter 9, Recognition of the Seriously Ill Child.

Respiratory rate and character

Breathing may be rapid and deep because of acidosis produced by poor tissue perfusion.

Mental status

Agitation and confusion may give way to increasing drowsiness and loss of consciousness. Infants may be drowsy but irritable with a weak cry and hypotonia.

Frequent reassessment is necessary to detect improvement or deterioration as early as possible

---

GENERAL MANAGEMENT OF SHOCK

1 Maintain a patent protected airway.
2 Ventilation (spontaneous or supported) should be given using 100% oxygen.
3 Venous or intraosseous access should be obtained. Central lines should be avoided.
4 20 ml/kg of crystalloid or colloid should be given immediately provided there is *evidence* of hypovolaemia or distributive shock (eg blood loss, history of severe diarrhoea and vomiting, rash of meningococcal sepsis).

SPECIFIC THERAPY OF SHOCK

Hypovolaemic shock

Hypovolaemia is the most common cause of shock in infancy and childhood and results from loss of circulating volume from any cause (Box 11.4). The keys to successful resuscitation are *early recognition* and *aggressive fluid replacement*.

Box 11.4 EXAMPLES OF CAUSES OF HYPOVOLAEMIC SHOCK

- Blood loss
    External haemorrhage, eg lacerations/open fractures
    Internal haemorrhage, eg ruptured spleen/closed fractures/gastrointestinal
- Loss of plasma
    Burns
- Dehydration
    Gastroenteritis
    Peritonitis
    Diabetes mellitus/insipidus
    Ileostomy losses

Transportation

Except in cases of entrapment, it will usually be possible to move the patient after stabilising the airway and breathing and a rapid circulatory assessment. It takes time to run through intravenous lines and site cannulae. These procedures can usually be done in transit, to minimise delay. ECG monitoring should be performed and vital signs documented. Frequent reassessment is necessary.

Fluid volume and type

- Fluids should be warmed if possible.
- An initial fluid bolus of 20 ml/kg of colloid or crystalloid (0.9% saline or Hartmanns solution) is given as fast as possible.
- This should be repeated after reassessment if there is no or inadequate improvement in vital signs.
- The most common mistake in the treatment of hypovolaemic shocked children is failure to give enough fluid.
- Further details on fluid administration can be found in Appendix A: Fluid administration.

Pitfalls in diagnosis

Hypovolaemic shock should never be attributed to an isolated head injury in a child, though rarely an infant may have an intracranial haematoma of sufficient volume to cause hypovolaemia. An infant with a patent fontanelle can lose a considerable volume of blood within the cranium as the cranium allows for expansion. In trauma, if hypovolaemia is unexplained, occult blood loss should be considered. This may be intraperitoneal, intrathoracic, around long bone or pelvic fractures, or retroperitoneal. Hypoglycaemia may give a similar clinical picture to that of compensated shock. This must always be excluded by urgent glucose stick test. Hypoglycaemia and hypovolaemia may coexist.

Distributive shock

Anaphylactic shock

Anaphylaxis is a potentially life threatening syndrome which may progress to shock. It is an immunologically mediated, generalised allergic reaction. The most common causes are allergy to penicillin, to radiographic contrast media, and to certain foods, especially nuts.

Prodromal symptoms of flushing, itching, facial swelling, urticaria, abdominal pain, diarrhoea, wheeze, and stridor may precede shock or may be the only manifestations of anaphylaxis. Symptoms and signs are shown in Table 11.5.

Treatment

Anaphylactic shock is caused by acute vasodilatation and by fluid loss from the intravascular space caused by increased capillary permeability. The allergen should be removed. Airway, breathing, and circulation should be assessed and high flow oxygen given.

The immediate further management centres on the administration of adrenaline and aggressive fluid resuscitation.

If the airway is completely obstructed, intubation will be necessary. Otherwise high flow oxygen should be given. Salbutamol should be administered via a nebuliser for wheeze. If there is evidence of circulatory compromise, the patient's ECG should be monitored, adrenaline 10 mcg/kg should be given intramuscularly and this should be followed by 20 ml/kg fluid (colloid or crystalloid). The adrenaline can be repeated every

Table 11.5. Symptoms and signs of anaphylactic shock

	Symptoms	Signs
Mild	Buming sensation in mouth Itching of lips, mouth, throat Feeling of warmth Nausea Abdominal pain	Urticarial rash Angio-oedema Conjunctivitis
Moderate +	Coughing/wheezing Loose bowel motions Sweating Irritability	Bronchospasm Tachycardia Pallor
Severe +	Difficulty breathing Collapse Vomiting Uncontrolled defecation	Severe bronchospasm Laryngeal oedema Shock Respiratory arrest Cardiac arrest

15 minutes until a satisfactory improvement is observed. The fluid challenge can also be repeated if required. Hydrocortisone 4 mg/kg and chlorpheniramine 0.2 mg/kg can also be given if available. Constant reassessment is essential.

Septic shock

Septic shock occurs because of a combination of complicated physiological events due primarily to circulating cytokines. These include vasodilatation and cardiac depression. Compensated septic shock may be difficult to diagnose because the extremities are warm and there may be a wide pulse pressure producing a hyperdynamic pulse. However, there will also be hyperpyrexia, hyperventilation, tachycardia, and mental confusion. If no effective therapy is given, cardiovascular performance will deteriorate and cardiac output diminishes. Even with a normal or raised cardiac output shock can develop. Hypotension may persist as a result of inappropriately decreased vascular resistance and capillary leakage. **Early aggressive therapy using volume replacement is crucial**.

Treatment

Airway and breathing   100% oxygen should be given. Ventilation may need to be supported using a bag and mask.

Circulation   The glucose stick should be checked on obtaining circulatory access as hypoglycaemia is common. Glucose levels <3 mmol/l should be treated with 5 ml/kg of 10% dextrose. Either crystalloid or colloid should be given in a bolus of 20 ml/kg and the patient reassessed. It may be necessary to repeat this until the circulation improves.

> **It is very important that hospital admission is not delayed in these children and intervention such as intravenous cannulation/intraosseous infusion should be initiated en route**

Disability   Initially, AVPU, posture and pupils must be documented. The conscious level should be monitored.

Secondary assessment   A careful examination for a meningococcal rash should be made and penicillin given if available (Table 10.3) if there is any suspicion of meningococcal sepsis and no history of allergy.

Cardiogenic shock

This is very rare and results from the causes listed in Table 11.2. It may be difficult to diagnose unless there is a clear history suggestive of it. Signs include those of heart failure, ie tachycardia, enlarged liver, and sweatiness, but these may be difficult to ascertain in the pre-hospital setting. If cardiogenic shock is suspected the patient should be given 100% oxygen and transported rapidly to hospital. A fluid bolus should **not** be given unless hypovolaemia is suspected, in which case **10 ml/kg** may be given cautiously over 2–5 minutes and the response assessed. If the child is much improved, consideration can be given for a further 10 ml/kg. If the child deteriorates, **STOP**.

Obstructive shock

The causes of obstructive shock are primarily traumatic and will be discussed later.

Dissociative shock

The main cause of dissociative shock to suspect in the pre-hospital setting is carbon monoxide poisoning. This is sometimes found in victims of burns and smoke inhalation. Faulty gas heating also may release carbon monoxide. A clue to the diagnosis may be the relative absence of cyanosis in the child in the presence of obvious severe respiratory failure. 100% oxygen should be given and rapid transportation to hospital undertaken. It may be necessary later to transfer the victim to a hyperbaric chamber where definitive oxygen therapy can be given. However, it will usually be necessary to confirm the diagnosis in a "normal" medical facility first. Pulse oximeters will not read accurately in a child with carbon monoxide poisoning.

NEUROLOGICAL PROBLEMS

CONVULSIONS

Glossary

Convulsion or seizure This is an abnormal paroxysmal discharge of cerebral neurones.

Febrile convulsions Children between the ages of 6 months and 6 years often develop a generalised tonic–clonic convulsion in response to a rapid rise in temperature. This is usually self-contained, stopping within 5–10 minutes. Provided the convulsion has stopped spontaneously and there has been no hypoxia, it is important to look for the cause of the fever.

Status epilepticus This occurs either when a convulsion lasts for longer than 30 minutes or when successive convulsions occur so frequently that the patient does not recover fully between them.

Tonic–clonic status is the most common form of status epilepticus. It occurs in approximately 1–5% of patients with epilepsy; 5–10% of children with febrile seizures will present in status epilepticus.

Status epilepticus can be fatal, although the mortality is higher in adults. Death may be due to complications of the convulsion, such as obstruction of the airway or aspiration of vomit, to overmedication, or to the underlying disease process.

Approximately two-thirds of children with status epilepticus that lasts longer than 60 minutes will have subsequent irreversible neurological handicaps. The incidence of neurological complications is higher in young infants. The common causes of status epilepticus are listed in Box 11.5.

Box 11.5 COMMONEST CAUSES OF STATUS EPILEPTICUS IN CHILDREN

- "Febrile" status epilepticus
- Sudden reduction in anti-epileptic medication
- Head injury
- Idiopathic epilepsy
- Meningitis
- Encephalopathy (including Reye's syndrome)
- Poisoning

Treatment of convulsions

Airway and breathing The airway may need clearing by suction. A Guedel airway or a nasopharyngeal airway may be required. 100% oxygen should be given via a non-rebreathing mask or alternatively if the patient is not breathing adequately, bag-and-mask ventilation may be required.

Circulation Establishing intravenous access in the first instance may slow transportation. A glucose stick test should be performed using a finger prick. If the blood glucose is <3 mmol/l glucose gel should be smeared round the patient's mouth whilst being careful to maintain the airway. If intravenous or intraosseous access is available, 5 ml/kg of 10% glucose can be given. A maximum concentration of 25% glucose is used in children (see section on Hypoglycaemia).

Disability 0.4 mg/kg diazepam should be administered rectally whilst the child is being transported (stop briefly to insert the tube). If the convulsion has not settled after 5 minutes this can be repeated once.

Additional treatment
Transportation should not be delayed if the child is still fitting. If the child feels very hot, clothing can be removed to cool him or her. The hospital should be advised of the patient's arrival if the child continues to convulse.

If a febrile convulsion has stopped by the time help arrives, the patient should still, as a minimum, be examined by a doctor to establish the cause of the fever. Generally however the parents will be very frightened and it is usual practice still to take the child to hospital. Frequently the child will be drowsy and in a post-ictal state. A blood glucose test is indicated, along with maintenance of the airway and breathing, and observation of vital signs.

COMA

Introduction

The conscious level may be altered by disease, injury, or intoxication. The level of awareness decreases as a child passes through stages from drowsiness (mild reduction in alertness and increase in hours of sleep) to unconsciousness (unrousable unresponsiveness). Because of variability in the definition of words describing the degree of coma, the Glasgow and the Children's Coma Scales have been developed as semiquantitative measures and, more importantly, as a communication aid between carers. The Glasgow Coma Scale has been validated whereas the Children's Coma Scale has not (Table 11.6).

Table 11.6. Coma scoring systems

Glasgow Coma Scale (4–15 years)		Children's Coma Scale (<4 years)		
Response	Score	Response		Score
Eyes		**Eyes**		
Open spontaneously	4	Open spontaneously		4
Verbal command	3	React to speech		3
Pain	2	React to pain		2
No response	1	No response		1
Best motor response		**Best motor response**		
Verbal command		Spontaneous or obeys verbal		
Obeys	6	command		6
Painful stimulus		*Painful stimulus*		
Localises pain	5	Localises pain		5
Flexion with pain	4	Withdraws in response to pain		4
Flexion abnormal	3	Abnormal flexion to pain		3
		(decorticate posture)		
Extension	2	Abnormal extension to pain		2
		(decerebrate posture)		
No response	1	No response		1
Best verbal response		**Best verbal response**		
Orientated and converses	5	Smiles, orientated to sounds, follows objects, interacts		5
		Crying	*Interacts*	
Disorientated and converses	4	Consolable	Inappropriate	4
Inappropriate words	3	Inconsistently consolable	Moaning	3
Incomprehensible sounds	2	Inconsolable	Irritable	2
No response	1	No response	No response	1

Pathophysiology and aetiology

Coma is a sign of significant "brain failure" and requires emergency treatment to prevent or minimise central nervous system damage.

In children, coma is caused by a diffuse metabolic insult (including cerebral hypoxia and ischaemia) in 95% of cases and by structural lesions in the remaining 5%. Metabolic disturbances can produce diffuse, incomplete, and asymmetrical neurological signs. Early signs may be subtle with reduced attention and blunted affect. The most common causes of coma are summarised in Box 11.6.

Treatment

The initial priority in the management of the unconscious child is the maintenance of airway, breathing, and circulation.

Airway   The airway should be cleared and a Guedel airway inserted if necessary. The cervical spine should be stabilised if there is any suspicion of trauma. Breathing and its adequacy should be assessed and 100% oxygen given.

> **Box 11.6 DISORDERS CAUSING COMA IN CHILDREN**
>
> Hypoxia—ischaemic brain injury
>   Following respiratory or circulatory failure
> Epileptic seizures
> Trauma
>   Intracranial haemorrhage, brain swelling
> Infections
>   Meningitis
>   Encephalitis
> Poisons
> Metabolic
>   Renal, hepatic failure, Reye's syndrome, hypoglycaemia, diabetes,
> hypothermia, hypercapnia
> Vascular lesions
>   Bleeding, arteriovenous malformations, arterial or venous thrombosis
> Hypertension

Breathing   Bag-valve-mask ventilation should be employed if breathing is inadequate. A saturation monitor should be attached if available.

Circulation   The circulation should be assessed in the usual way and shock treated appropriately. A glucose stick should be performed and if the blood sugar is <3 mmol/l, hypoglycaemia should be treated, either with glucose gel or with 5 ml/kg of 10% glucose by the intravenous or intraosseous routes.

"Treat the treatable"

If the child is stable with regard to cardiorespiratory function, specific conditions should then be sought and treated on the way to hospital.

1   Hypoglycaemia as outlined above.
2   Poisoning with opiates—naloxone 10 mcg/kg intravenously followed by 100 mcg/kg intramuscularly.
3   Meningococcal septicaemia, as outlined in the section on septic shock and Table 10.3.

A rapid assessment of disability should be made using AVPU and pupil assessment.

History

A more detailed history should be taken, including any history of recent trauma, epilepsy, ingestion of poisons, and chronic conditions. The time when the patient last ate should be noted and recent trips abroad documented. Any known chronic condition should also be documented.

If there is time during the transport to hospital, a Glasgow coma score or Children's coma score can be performed and a rapid general physical assessment should be made, looking for signs of a purpuric rash, any injuries, enlarged liver or underlying conditions (such as the presence of a ventriculoperitoneal shunt for hydrocephalus).

The hospital should be warned of the child's condition and the child monitored for deterioration.

Coma that develops slowly over a period of hours or days is usually due to an infection (meningitis/encephalitis), a metabolic disturbance, Reye's syndrome or a mass lesion. Sudden onset suggests an epileptic seizure, poisoning or, more rarely, a vascular event.

Previous episodes of coma suggest certain inborn errors of metabolism or endocrine disease such as diabetes, epilepsy, porphyria or repeated poisoning.

> **Danger signs in the child with coma include:**
>
> - Glasgow coma score <8
> - Glasgow coma score dropping
> - Development of unequal pupils
> - Rising blood pressure and slowing pulse

HYPOGLYCAEMIA

Hypoglycaemia in children is relatively common and may be due to:

- Diabetes mellitus.
- Poor liver reserves of glucose (eg any seriously ill child, pre-term babies).
- Metabolic abnormality.

Treatment

All children who have an impaired conscious level must have their airway, breathing, and circulation maintained in the usual way.

If the child is conscious, glucose or glucose gel can be administered. If unconscious, glucose gel can be smeared around the child's mouth whilst being careful to maintain the airway. If this is ineffective, glucagon can be given intramuscularly whilst in transit. This treatment is likely to be effective in diabetics as glucagon mobilises glucose from the liver. In children with other causes of hypoglycaemia, it is much less likely to work as most of their stores are already used up. If glucagon fails, intravenous or intraosseous glucose should be given at a dose of 5 ml/kg of 10% dextrose as a bolus titrated to a response. (Half the volume of 20% dextrose may also be used.) If the child already has intravenous access, intravenous glucose may be used as the first choice therapy.

> **50% glucose should never be given to children as it has been known to cause cerebral oedema and death**

POISONING

Poisoning in young children is common, and accounts for about 20 000 hospital admissions per year. The numbers have dropped since the introduction of child resistant containers, but it must be remembered that 20% of children under the age of 5 can open these.

Aetiology

Accidental poisoning This is usually a problem of the young child or toddler, with a mean age of presentation of $2\frac{1}{2}$ years. Accidental poisoning usually occurs when the child is unsupervised, and there is an increased incidence in poisoning following recent disruption in households, such as a new baby, moving house, or where there is maternal depression. Paracetamol, antibiotics, iron tablets, and the oral contraceptive pill are particularly commonly ingested.

Intentional overdose Suicide or parasuicide attempts are usually made by young people in their teens. These children or adolescents should be admitted to hospital and undergo full psychiatric and social assessment.

Drug abuse Alcohol and solvent abuse are the most common forms of drug abuse in children in the UK.

Iatrogenic The most frequently fatal drug is digoxin.

Deliberate poisoning Rarely, symptoms are induced in children by adults by the administration of drugs. A history of poisoning will often not be given at presentation.

Presentation

History

What? Ask accompanying adults to bring the container to hospital, with its remaining contents, or specimen of berries or plants that have been eaten. Take careful note of trade names and all constituents of anything that might have been ingested, as the local poisons unit will need all the details in order to provide the correct advice to the hospital.

How much? Assume the worst, so if ten tablets are missing assume the child has eaten them all.

When? This is important for the hospital to know, in order to determine the timing of blood levels, and to decide about appropriate treatments such as stomach-emptying procedures.

Has the child vomited? If so, has any of the vomit been retained for inspection and possible tablet analysis? If it is possible to do so, a sample should be brought to hospital.

Why? Was the poisoning accidental, and if so how could it have been avoided? Remember non-accidental injury.

Absent history? Always suspect poisoning in any child with signs that cannot otherwise be explained, especially the following:

- Drowsiness or coma.
- Convulsions.
- Tachypnoea.
- Tachycardia or flushing.
- Cardiac arrhythmia or hypotension.
- Unusual behaviour.
- Pupillary abnormalities.

Various drugs cause specific signs when taken in overdose and thus clues as to the drug ingested may be found in the primary and secondary assessment. These signs are summarised in Table 11.7.

Full and careful examination of the child should follow the ABCD protocol with resuscitative measures as appropriate; remember to record vital signs such as respiratory and pulse rate, blood pressure, and conscious level.

Management

Airway and breathing The airway must be maintained in the usual way and 100% oxygen should be given unless paraquat poisoning is suspected, in which case advice from the Poisons Information Centre should be taken. If breathing is inadequate bag-valve-mask ventilation may be required. Oxygen saturation should be monitored where possible.

Table 11.7. Signs of specific poisonings

Signs	Drug
Tachypnoea	Aspirln, theophylline, carbon monoxide, cyanide
Bradypnoea	Ethanol, opiates, barbiturates, sedatives
Metabolic acidosis (sighing respirations)	Ethanol, carbon monoxide, ethylene glycol
Tachycardia	Antidepressants, sympathomimetics, amphetamines, cocaine
Bradycardia	β-blockers, digoxin, clonidine
Hypotension	Barbiturates, benzodiazepines, β-blockers, calcium channel blockers, opiates, iron, phenothiazines, phenytoin, tricyclic antidepressants
Hypertension	Amphetamines, cocaine, sympathomimetic agents
Small pupils	Opiates, organophosphate insecticides, phenothiazines
Large pupils	Amphetamines, atropine, cannabis, carbamazepine, cocaine, quinine, tricyclic antidepressants
Convulsions	Carbamazepine, lindane organophosphate insecticides, phenothiazines, tricyclic antidepressants
Hypothermia	Barbiturates, ethanol, phenothiazines
Hyperthermia	Amphetamines, cocaine, Ecstasy, phenothiazines, salicylates

Circulation   This should be assessed in the usual way and ECG monitoring should be performed. A number of poisons produce shock, in addition to those substances which cause arrhythmias. Consider cannulation en route in those at high risk from arrhythmias.

Disability   AVPU and pupils should be checked. Convulsions should be controlled in the usual way.

Specific treatments   Do not induce vomiting. Most specific treatments are not practical in the pre-hospital setting. However, the treatment of possible *opiate poisoning* (such as methadone) is not only practical but easy. If there is any possibility that *opiates* have been given the child should be treated with naloxone. This can be given intramuscularly and it is therefore not necessary to delay transport by obtaining intravenous access. If you are some distance from a hospital remember that the half-life of the opiate may be longer than that of naloxone and further doses may be required. *Carbon monoxide poisoning* (see "Dissociative shock" above) is treated with as high a percentage oxygen as can be obtained. Pulse oximetry is not reliable in carbon monoxide poisoning.

Transport   The child should be moved to hospital as soon as possible, together with the container, berries, plants, remaining tablets etc. Identification of toxins has recently become easier with a new CD-ROM which can display "pictures" of poisonous substances/plants.

SUMMARY

Treatment of medical conditions follows ABCD.

- Respiratory conditions account for 30–40% of hospital admissions and about 450 children per year will die because of them.
- In upper airway obstruction—do no harm!
- Salbutamol is indicated for lower airway obstruction (wheeze).
- Early recognition of shock and appropriate management **of the cause** is vital.
- Children with meningococcal septicaemia should receive penicillin and supportive therapy as soon as possible.
- In coma and convulsions "treat the treatable" after ABC.
- 50% dextrose should not be used to treat hypoglycaemia in children.
- All children with serious medical problems should be transferred to hospital as soon as possible.

Questions

1 What is the most important part of the management of a child with viral croup who is able to breathe?

2 Approximately what percentage blood has been lost in an 8-year-old child who has tachycardia, is lethargic, and has a systolic blood pressure of 80 mmHg?

3 List the *specific* drug treatments for the following:
   (a) meningococcal septicaemia
   (b) opiate poisoning
   (c) anaphylactic shock
   (d) wheezing
   (e) carbon monoxide poisoning.

4 How should dissociative shock be treated? Give one cause of dissociative shock

5 List four conditions where pulse oximetry may be unreliable.

12

The structured approach to the seriously injured child

OBJECTIVES

After reading this chapter you should be able to:

- Identify the physical signs assessed in the primary survey
- Describe the possible treatment a traumatised child may require during resuscitation
- Recognise the abnormalities which may be found in the secondary survey
- Describe the importance of note taking and adequate handover at hospital

---

INTRODUCTION

This chapter sets out a structured approach to the initial assessment and management of the seriously injured child. It is essential that the scene has been assessed and deemed safe before the management of injuries can begin. Children and adults are affected quite differently by major injuries physically, physiologically, and psychologically. A young child cannot describe pain, or even localise symptoms. The more frightened children become the "younger" they may behave, and the less they can contribute to management. They may even deny *all* symptoms vehemently.

Often these difficulties are compounded by the rescuers' perception of the child's vulnerability and the need to provide "**better**" care to the injured child. This may lead to rushed decision making which has an emotional rather than clinical basis.

Although traumatised children have a number of unique problems this in no way affects the validity of a structured approach. Additional complicating factors found in the pre-hospital setting, such as the environment, eagerness of others on scene, weather conditions, and lack of exposure to traumatised children reinforces the need for a structured approach. By following the principles outlined in this chapter, problems will be identified and treated in order of priority. It should be emphasised from the start that, although assessment and management are discussed separately, this is purely to allow clarity. When dealing with an injured child it is essential that appropriate resuscitative measures are taken as soon as a problem is found.

The structured approach

Primary survey
Resuscitation
Alert and transfer to definitive care
Secondary survey (where appropriate)
Emergency treatment

PRIMARY SURVEY

During the primary survey life threatening conditions are identified. Assessment follows the familiar ABC pattern with significant additions:

> **A** **A**irway and *cervical spine control*
> **B** **B**reathing
> **C** **C**irculation and *haemorrhage control*
> **D** **D**isability
> **E** **E**xposure

Airway and cervical spine

Manual immobilisation of the cervical spine should be implemented immediately and the airway assessed for signs of obstruction:

- **LOOK** for obvious debris, cyanosis, agitation and obtundation.
- **LISTEN** for noisy breathing, including stridor or hoarseness.
- **FEEL** for movement of air during expiration and assess for tracheal deviation.

A cervical spine injury should be assumed to be present until adequate investigations have taken place in hospital.

Breathing

Once the airway has been secured and the cervical spine controlled, breathing should be assessed. As discussed in earlier chapters, the adequacy of breathing is gained from three sets of observations:

- The "work of breathing".
- The effectiveness of breathing.
- The effects of inadequate respiration on other organ systems.

These are summarised in Box 12.1.

> **Box 12.1 ASSESSMENT OF THE ADEQUACY OF BREATHING**
>
> - **The work of breathing**
>
>   Recession
>   Respiratory rate
>   Inspiratory or expiratory noises
>   Grunting
>   Accessory muscle use
>   Alae nasi flare
>
> - **Effectiveness of breathing**
>
>   Breath sounds
>   Chest expansion
>   Abdominal excursion
>
> - **Effects of inadequate respiration**
>
>   Heart rate
>   Skin colour
>   Mental status

The normal resting respiratory rate changes with age. An infant will take 40 breaths per minute, a pre-school child 30, and an adolescent 20.

Circulation

Circulation assessment in the primary survey consists of the rapid assessment of heart rate, capillary refill time, skin colour and temperature, respiratory rate, and mental status. Using these measures an approximate estimate of the percentage of blood loss can be made as shown in Table 12.1. When assessing circulatory status, allowance should be made for environmental conditions such as weather and lighting, which may affect the reliability of these signs.

Table 12.1. Recognition of stages of shock

	Compensated	Uncompensated	Pre-terminal (? irreversible)
Percentage blood loss	Up to 25	25–40	Over 40
Heart rate	Tachycardia +	Tachycardia + +	Tachycardia/ bradycardia
Systolic BP	Normal	Normal or falling	Falling
Pulse volume	Normal/reduced	Reduced +	Reduced + +
Capillary refill time (Normal <2 s)	Normal/increased	Increased +	Increased + +
Skin	Cool, pale	Cold, mottled	Cold, pale
Respiratory rate	Tachypnoea +	Tachypnoea + +	Sighing respiration
Mental state	Mild agitation	Lethargic Uncooperative	Reacts only to pain

Resting heart rate, blood pressure, and respiratory rate vary with age, and circulatory assessment of a child must take this variation into account. The normal values are shown in Table 12.2.

Table 12.2. Vital signs: approximate range of normal

Age (years)	Respiratory rate (breaths/min)	Systolic BP (mmHg)	Pulse (beats/min)
<1	30–40	70–90	110–160
2–5	25–30	80–100	95–140
5–12	20–25	90–110	80–120
>12	15–20	100–120	60–100

Disability

The assessment of disability during the primary survey consists of a brief neurological examination to determine conscious level and assessment of pupil size and reactivity. Conscious level determination is kept as simple as possible—and requires only that the child is put into one of the four following categories:

A ALERT
V responds to VOICE
P responds to PAIN
U UNRESPONSIVE

Exposure

In order to assess an injured child fully, it is necessary to remove his or her clothes. Children become cold very quickly due to their relatively large surface area, and may also be acutely embarrassed when undressed in front of strangers. The need for exposure in the pre-hospital setting will vary depending on the child's overall condition and should initially be restricted to the identification of an injury or condition. Exposure must be undertaken in a warm environment without unnecessary distress to the child.

RESUSCITATION

> **Life threatening problems should be treated as they are identified during the primary survey**

Airway and cervical spine

Airway

The airway may be compromised by extrinsic material (blood, vomit, or a foreign body), by the tongue, or by injury to the face, mouth, or upper airway. Whatever the cause, airway management should follow the sequence described in Chapter 7. This is summarised in Box 12.2 below.

> **Box 12.2 AIRWAY MANAGEMENT SEQUENCE**
> - Jaw thrust
> - Suction/removal of foreign body
> - Oropharyngeal airway
> - Endotracheal intubation
> - Surgical airway

Head tilt/chin lift is not recommended following trauma, because cervical spine injuries may be made worse.

Cervical spine

The cervical spine should be presumed to be damaged until proved intact, especially if there is obvious injury above the clavicle. If the child is unconscious or cooperative the head and neck should be immobilised initially with in-line manual stabilisation and then using a semi-rigid collar and appropriate immobilisation system. Uncooperative or combative patients should simply have a semi-rigid collar applied, since too rigid immobilisation of the head may increase neck movement as struggling occurs. Immobilising manoeuvres must be maintained throughout the care of the patient.

Breathing

If breathing is inadequate, ventilation must be commenced. Initially bag-and-mask ventilation should be performed. Intubation should only be considered following failure to achieve adequate oxygenation via the bag-and-mask technique. It is often impractical outside hospital if the patient is breathing, because of the need for general anaesthetic.

If breath sounds are unequal then pneumothorax, misplaced endotracheal tube, or blocked main bronchus should be considered and appropriate measures taken.

Circulation

A seriously injured child may require urgent establishment of vascular access. This should be established while en route to hospital, and fluid therapy initiated as detailed in Appendix A. A trapped child may require fluids at the scene.

The percutaneous approach to peripheral veins using a large bore cannula is the preferred route, but, if this fails, intraosseous infusion should be used.

Relevant history

The mechanism of injury may be useful. The information in Table 12.3 should be obtained if possible and included within the written report to the receiving hospital.

Table 12.3. Relevant history

Road accident	Other
Car occupant/cyclist/pedestrian	Nature of accident
Position in vehicle	Objects involved
Restraints worn	Height of fall
Head protection	Landing surface
Thrown from vehicle	Environmental (temperature,
Speed of impact	contamination)
Damage to the vehicle	
Other victims' injuries	
Deaths in vehicle	

Analgesia

Analgesia should be considered at this stage and administered unless there is very good reason for not doing so. Morphine is the drug of choice and should be given intravenously in a dose of 0.1 mg/kg. There is no place for the administration of intramuscular analgesia in trauma. Entonox (a 50/50 mix of O_2/N_2O) should be considered, but is contraindicated if there is a possibility of pneumothorax or base of skull fracture.

SECONDARY SURVEY

Head-to-toe examination

If no life threatening conditions are found then a brief secondary survey may be undertaken, preferably in the warm environment of the ambulance en route to hospital. This secondary survey must not delay transportation or cause distress to the child. If any life threatening problems are found during this survey, it must be abandoned, the problem dealt with, and urgent transportation continued. The secondary survey will usually be performed after arrival in hospital.

Head

- Inspect for bruising, lacerations, haemorrhage, deformity and CSF leak.
- Palpate for lacerations, bruising, and skull depressions.
- Perform otoscopy and ophthalmoscopy (if equipment available).
- Perform mini-neurological examination:
    pupillary reflexes;
    Glasgow Coma Score;
    motor functions.

Face

- Inspect for bruising, lacerations, and deformity.
- Inspect the mouth, inside and out.

101

- Palpate the bones for deformity.
- Palpate the teeth for looseness.

Neck

Care should be taken not to move the cervical spine during this assessment. If the semi-rigid collar is removed, an assistant should maintain in-line cervical stabilisation throughout.

- Inspect the front and back of the neck for bruising and swelling:
- Palpate for surgical emphysema.

Chest

- Inspect for bruising, lacerations, deformity, and movement.
- Inspect neck veins.
- Feel for tenderness, crepitus, and paradoxical movement.
- Feel for tracheal deviation.
- Percuss the chest wall.
- Listen for breath sounds and added sounds.
- Listen for heart sounds.

Abdomen

- Observe for movement.
- Inspect for bruising, lacerations, and swelling.
- Palpate for tenderness, rigidity, and masses.
- Auscultate for bowel sounds.

Pelvis

- Inspect for bruising, lacerations, and deformity.
- The pelvis should not be repeatedly palpated if a fracture is suspected as a clot may be dislodged internally and bleeding worsened.

Back/Spine

Proper examination of the spine can only be carried out after the child has been log-rolled and should ideally only be performed in the hospital. If there is a suspicion of injury to this area which may require immediate attention, ie major bleeding, then it may be necessary to examine the back area while on the scene.

Extremities

- Observe for bruising, swelling, and deformity.
- Palpate for tenderness. Crepitus and abnormal movement may be found (do not elicit deliberately as these are painful).
- Assess peripheral circulation—pulses and capillary return.
- Assess peripheral sensation—to touch.

EMERGENCY TREATMENT

This is treatment which is necessary during the first hour or so of management, and this may occasionally be carried out before arrival at hospital. These procedures are not as urgent as those performed to save life during resuscitation but are important nevertheless. Once the secondary survey is completed an emergency treatment plan can be formulated. This will include treatments for potentially life threatening and limb threatening injuries discovered during the secondary survey and for more minor injuries discovered at the same time. They will be discussed in more detail in the next chapter.

CONTINUED MONITORING DURING TRANSPORTATION

Pulse, capillary refill time, respiratory rate, pupil size and reactivity, and Glasgow Coma Score should be measured and charted frequently (at least every 15 minutes). Blood pressure may be taken if logistics allow. Oxygen saturation provides useful additional information, and should be measured if possible.

Any deterioration should lead to immediate reassessment of the airway, breathing, and circulation, and appropriate resuscitative measures should be commenced.

DEFINITIVE CARE

Definitive care cannot be achieved in the pre-hospital setting and this must be remembered when considering any intervention. Any intervention performed in transit will delay definitive care and must be justified by the need to provide immediate resuscitation.

Patient reporting/handover

The structured approach discussed in this chapter can provide a framework for the writing of notes. It is recommended that these should be set out as shown in Box 12.3.

Box 12.3 TEMPLATE FOR NOTE TAKING

- **History**

- **Primary survey**

    A
    B
    C
    D
    E

- **Resuscitation**

    A
    B
    C

- **Secondary survey**

    Head
    Face
    Neck
    Chest
    Abdomen
    Pelvis
    Spine
    Extremities
    Upper
    Lower

ALERTING THE HOSPITAL

It is essential that all relevant information is passed to the receiving hospital as soon as possible.

The hospital may need to alert specialist staff or make facilities available to treat the child. Alerting the receiving hospital with appropriate information will prevent unnecessary delay on arrival and may be the difference between a good and bad outcome (Box 4.1, "ASHICE").

SUMMARY

The structured approach to initial assessment and management discussed here allows the health professional to care for the seriously injured child in a logical, efficacious fashion.

Assessment of vital functions (airway, breathing, and circulation) is carried out first; resuscitation for any problems found is instituted immediately.

- Primary survey.
- Resuscitation.

During transportation

- Monitor vital signs and reassess constantly.
- Continue resuscitation (eg vascular access, etc).
- Secondary survey (if appropriate).
- Emergency treatment.

Questions

1 Name six physical signs which are useful in the assessment of shock.
2 What treatments or manoeuvres may be required to secure the airway and in which order would they be attempted?
3 What are the four "modes" of examination when examining the patient during the secondary survey?

13

Treating seriously injured children

This chapter has been divided into three sections:

Section 1
Trauma to the head and spine

Section 2
Trauma to the chest and abdomen

Section 3
Trauma to the extremities, burns, electrical injuries, and near drowning

13.1

Trauma to the head and spine

> **OBJECTIVES**
>
> After reading this section you should be able to:
>
> - Identify causes of primary and secondary brain damage.
> - State the factors indicating a potentially serious head injury.
> - Describe the assessment and resuscitation of a child with trauma to the head
> - State the factors indicating suspected spinal trauma
> - Describe the assessment and resuscitation of a child with suspected spinal injury

HEAD TRAUMA

Epidemiology

> **Head injury is the commonest single cause of death in children aged 1–15 years. It accounts for 15% of deaths in this age group, and for 25% of deaths in the 5–15 year age group**

The most common cause of death from head injury is a road traffic accident. Pedestrian children are the most vulnerable, followed by cyclists, and then passengers in vehicles. Falls are the second commonest cause of fatal head injuries, while in infancy the commonest mechanism is child abuse.

Pathophysiology

Brain damage may be from the primary or secondary effects of the injury.

Primary injury

Primary injury occurs at the time of impact and may be due to blunt or penetrating trauma and includes:

- Cerebral lacerations.
- Cerebral contusions.
- Dural sac tears.
- Diffuse axonal injury.

Secondary injury

This may result from either the secondary effects of cerebral injury or from the cerebral consequences of associated injuries and stress.

These may be due to:

- Hypoxia from inadequate ventilation caused by loss of respiratory drive.
- Hypoxia from airway obstruction or thoracic injuries.
- Ischaemia from poor cerebral perfusion secondary to raised intracranial pressure.
- Ischaemia secondary to hypotension and blood loss.
- Hypoglycaemia or other metabolic abnormality.
- Hypothermia.
- Fever.
- Convulsions.

Raised intracranial pressure

Once the sutures of the skull have closed at 12–18 months of age the child's cranial cavity behaves like an adult's, with a fixed volume. Cerebral oedema or haematomas increase that volume, but there are initial compensatory mechanisms, eg a reduction of the total volume of CSF and the pool of venous blood. When these mechanisms fail, the volume increase leads to a rapid rise in intracranial pressure. This causes an increased pressure gradient for the inflow of arterial blood and a consequent fall in cerebral perfusion pressure:

cerebral perfusion pressure = mean systemic BP – mean intracranial pressure

Normal cerebral perfusion is 50 ml of blood per 100 g brain tissue per minute. A fall in cerebral perfusion pressure decreases cerebral blood flow. A flow of below 20 ml per 100 g of brain tissue per minute will produce ischaemia; this increases cerebral oedema and hence causes a further rise in intracranial pressure. A cerebral blood flow of below 10 ml per 100 g per minute leads to electrical dysfunction of the neurones and loss of intracellular homeostasis.

A generalised increase of intracranial pressure in the supratentorial compartment initially causes transtentorial herniation, and later causes transforaminal herniation (coning) and death. Unilateral increases in intracranial pressure secondary to haematoma formation cause ipsilateral uncal herniation. The third nerve is nipped against the free border of the tentorium causing ipsilateral pupillary dilatation secondary to loss of parasympathetic constrictor tone to the ciliary muscles (Figure 13.1).

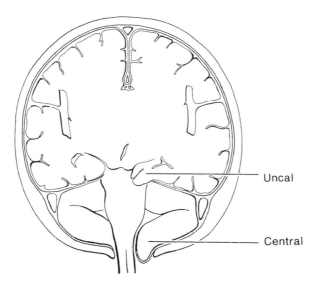

Uncal

Central

Figure 13.1. Herniation of the brain

107

In childhood, the commonest cause of raised intracranial pressure following head injury is cerebral oedema. Children are especially prone to this problem. They may, of course, also have expanding extradural, subdural or intracerebral haematomas which will require surgical treatment.

Depending on the aetiology of the raised intracranial pressure definitive treatment is either aimed at preventing further rises, or removing their causes (by surgical evacuation of haematomas).

There are special considerations in infants with head injuries. Their cranial volumes can more easily increase because of unfused sutures. Therefore, large extradural or subdural bleeds may occur before neurological signs or symptoms show. Additionally, the infant's vascular scalp may bleed profusely causing shock. In children over 1 year, shock associated with head injury means serious extracranial injury.

Head injuries vary from the trivial to the fatal. Factors indicating a potentially serious injury are shown in Box 13.1.

Box 13.1 FACTORS INDICATING A POTENTIALLY SERIOUS INJURY

- Mechanism of injury suggesting substantial force
- A history of loss of consciousness
- Children who are not fully conscious and responsive
- Any child with obvious neurological signs/symptoms
- Convulsions or limb weakness
- Evidence of penetrating injury to the head

Assessment

Primary survey

The first priority is to assess and stabilise the airway with cervical spine immobilisation, breathing, and circulation as discussed in Chapter 12. Remember that head injury may be associated with cervical spine injury and therefore neck immobilisation must be achieved.

An increase in intracranial pressure will cause a change in both respiratory rate and pattern, which may result in apnoea if not adequately treated during the primary assessment. The pulse may also be affected by an increase in intracranial pressure resulting in a bradycardia with an associated increase in systolic blood pressure.

Pupil size and reactivity should be examined, and a rapid assessment of conscious level should be made. The latter consists of assessing the disability of the child into one of four categories (AVPU).

Alert
Responds only to **V**oice
Responds only to **P**ain
Unresponsive

The history of the injury itself and the child's course since the injury occurred should be established from relevant personnel. Any other significant history may be obtained from parents or carers.

Resuscitation

The initial aim of management of a child with a serious head injury is prevention of secondary brain damage. This is achieved by maintaining ventilation and circulation, and by avoiding raised intracranial pressure.

Analgesia

Withholding analgesia may contribute to a deterioration of the child's condition by leading to a rise in intracranial pressure, and may lead to misinterpretation of the conscious level. Following initial assessment, sufficient analgesia should be administered. Entonox should not be given in case a basal skull fracture is present. Analgesia available may include morphine and nalbuphine. Ketamine should be avoided if the intracranial pressure may be raised.

Management of specific problems

Deteriorating conscious level   If airway, breathing, and circulation are satisfactory then a deteriorating conscious level should be assumed to be due to increased intracranial pressure. This may either be due to an intracranial haematoma or cerebral oedema. Mild hyperventilation should be considered as a temporising manoeuvre until arrival at hospital.

Convulsions   A focal seizure should be regarded as a focal neurological sign. A generalised convulsion has less significance. Seizure activity raises intracranial pressure. Seizures should be controlled if they have not stopped spontaneously within 5 minutes. An appropriate dose of diazepam should be given.

Secondary survey

The head should be carefully observed for injury and palpated for lacerations to the scalp and for depressed skull fractures. Look for evidence of basal skull fracture such as blood or CSF from the nose or ear, racoon eyes or Battle's sign (bruising behind the ear, over the mastoid), which is unlikely to be seen as it takes a number of hours to develop.

The conscious level should be assessed using the Children's Coma Scale if the child is less than 4, or the Glasgow Coma Scale if the child is older. It should be noted that the coma scales reflect the degree of brain dysfunction *at the time of the examination*. Reassessment should therefore be frequent (see Table 11.6).

The pupils should be examined for size and reactivity. A dilated non-reactive pupil indicates third nerve dysfunction, the usual cause being an ipsilateral haematoma. The side of the dilated pupil should be carefully documented.

SPINAL TRAUMA

Spinal injuries are rare in children. That does not mean they are unimportant. A high index of suspicion, correct management, and prompt referral are necessary in order to prevent exacerbation of underlying cord injury. **All severely injured children should be treated as though they have spinal injury until adequate examination and investigation excludes it.**

Injuries of the cervical spine

The upper three vertebrae are usually involved in children, while in adults injury to the lower segments is commoner. The low incidence (0.2% of all children's fractures and dislocations) of bony injury is explained by the mobility of the cervical spine in children, which dissipates applied forces over a greater number of segments.

Injuries of the thoracic and lumbar spine

Injuries to the thoracic and lumbar spine are rare in children and account for less than 1% of all spinal injuries. They are most common in the multiply injured child. In the second decade, 44% of reported injuries may result from sporting and other recreational activity. Some spinal injuries may result from non-accidental injury.

When an injury does occur it is not uncommon to find multiple levels of involvement since the force is dissipated over many segments in the child's mobile spine. This increased mobility may also lead to neurological involvement without significant skeletal injury.

If cord damage does occur, children can suffer the same complications as adults. In addition, late, progressive deformity to the spine may occur secondary to differential growth occurring around the injured segments.

Assessment

The most common mechanism of injury is hyperflexion. Because of the difficulties of assessment the history of the accident may be the only indication to suspect a spinal injury. A child who has fallen, who has multiple injuries or has been involved in any accident where force has been applied, should be suspected of having a spinal injury and should be immobilised on a long spine board until investigations and examinations are completed in hospital.

Primary survey

The primary assessment of a child who is suspected of having spinal trauma should follow an assessment of the airway with immobilisation of the cervical spine as described in Chapter 16, followed by assessment of breathing, circulation, and disability. Care must be taken to protect the spine throughout the assessment and treatment of the child.

Further to a history of applied force, indications of spinal injury may also include:

- Back or neck pain at rest or during movement.
- Tenderness over the spine.
- Pain during palpation.
- Deformity or swelling.
- Guarding of the neck or back.
- Paralysis.
- Numbness.
- Tingling or "pins and needles".

> Despite the rarity of fractures, a severely injured child's spine should be securely immobilised until orthopaedic or neurosurgical advice has been obtained in hospital

Children frequently become frightened during spinal immobilisation and may become combative. Appropriate explanation and reassurance may be all that is required to prevent this. In other cases, it may not be possible to tape the head during cervical spine immobilisation and a child may even refuse to have a collar fitted. In these cases, manual immobilisation is the best and safest alternative as forced attempts with a collar and tape may cause further damage. Once a child has been immobilised, ensure that you are within his or her line of vision when talking to them. This will prevent the child naturally trying to twist the head. Parents should also be specifically instructed to do this when reassuring their child.

It may be difficult to distinguish between a combative, frightened child and a genuinely confused child with a head injury—never become impatient in this situation.

Resuscitation

Treatment following suspected spinal injury follows the same priorities of airway with cervical immobilisation, breathing, circulation, and disability—as with all other injuries. Life threatening problems must be treated as they are found and will indicate the need for rapid removal of the child to hospital. Remember, spinal cord injury can lead to distributive shock. The presence of suspected spinal trauma in these situations should not delay the removal of the child to hospital. Teamwork will be required to ensure that this is undertaken without compromise to the spine. As with all transfers, the hospital must be alerted and kept updated as necessary.

Consideration should be given to the use of police to help progress to hospital by providing an escort for the ambulance or supervising traffic junctions if this is felt to be necessary.

SUMMARY

Head injury

- Head injury causes primary brain damage. Secondary damage primarily occurs because of the effects of hypoxia and poor cerebral perfusion.
- Factors present that may indicate a serious head injury include loss of consciousness, neurological signs, and weakness.
- The first priority is assessment and management of the airway with cervical spine immobilisation, breathing, circulation, and rapid assessment of conscious level using AVPU.
- A thorough examination and a mini-neurological examination should be carried out during the secondary survey. This involves a more detailed assessment of external injury, conscious level, and pupillary responses.

Spinal injury

- Spinal injuries are rare in children and are most commonly caused by hyperflexion.
- The first priority is assessment and management of the airway with cervical spine immobilisation, breathing, circulation, and rapid assessment of conscious level using AVPU.
- The most important indication of spinal injury is a history of force to the child.
- All children with suspected spinal injury should have their spine fully immobilised until such time as orthopaedic or neurological advice has been obtained in hospital.

Questions

1 List three possible causes of *primary* brain injury.
2 List three factors indicating a potentially serious head injury.
3 What is the most important indicator of potential spinal injury?
4 List four other factors indicating a potential spinal trauma.

SECTION

13.2

Trauma to the chest and abdomen

OBJECTIVES

After reading this section you should be able to:

- State the serious injuries which may result following chest and abdominal trauma
- Describe the assessment and resuscitation of a child with chest trauma
- Describe the assessment and resuscitation of a child with abdominal trauma

---

CHEST TRAUMA

Following the establishment of a secure airway, the next consideration in the resuscitation of a child is the assessment of breathing. The child who has suffered multiple injuries may well have significant intrathoracic trauma that severely compromises respiration, and may require immediate treatment.

Due to the soft compliant chest wall, substantial amounts of kinetic energy may be transferred through a child's chest wall with little or no external sign of injury.

Rib fractures over flail segments are very rare in children because of their compliant chests, but children may develop pulmonary contusions or pneumothoraces with apparently very little external injury. Because of the mobility of children's organs within the mediastinum, tension pneumothorax may develop more quickly than with adults.

Thoracic injuries must be considered in all children who suffer major trauma. Some may be life threatening and require immediate therapy during the primary survey and resuscitation, while others may be discovered during the secondary survey.

Practical trauma procedures are described in detail in Chapter 16.

Assessment: injuries posing an immediate threat to life

Tension pneumothorax

In this condition air accumulates under pressure in the pleural space. This pushes the mediastinum across the chest and kinks the great vessels in the mediastinum. This, in turn, impedes venous return to the heart resulting in a reduced cardiac output. The diagnosis is a clinical one.

Signs
- The child will be hypoxic and may be shocked.
- There will be decreased air entry and hyper-resonance to percussion on the side of the pneumothorax.

112

- Distended neck veins may be apparent in thin children.
- The trachea will be deviated away from the side of the pneumothorax (late sign).

Resuscitation
- High concentration oxygen should be given through a reservoir mask.
- Immediate needle thoracocentesis should be performed to relieve the tension (see Chapter 16).
- Air may be forced into any pneumothorax by artificial ventilation. A patient with a simple pneumothorax will develop a tension pneumothorax if ventilated.

Massive haemopneumothorax

In this condition, air and blood accumulates in the pleural space. This usually results from damage to the lung parenchyma with possible additional damage to pulmonary or chest wall blood vessels. The haemothorax can contain a substantial proportion of the child's blood volume, resulting in hypotension and compounding the reduced ventilatory state.

Signs
- The child will be hypoxic and shocked.
- There will be:
    decreased chest movement on the affected side;
    decreased air entry on the affected side;
    decreased resonance to percussion on the side of the haemopneumothorax.

Resuscitation
- High flow oxygen should be given through a reservoir mask.
- IV access should be attempted and volume replacement commenced if appropriate.
- The hospital should be alerted and the child transferred urgently.

Open pneumothorax

This occurs when there is a penetrating wound in the chest wall with an associated pneumothorax. The wound may be obvious, but it may be on the patient's back, and then will not be seen unless actively looked for.

Air may be heard sucking and blowing through the wound. The other signs of pneumothorax will be present, including:

- Decreased chest movement on the affected side.
- Decreased air entry on the affected side.
- Increased resonance to percussion on the side of the pneumothorax.

Resuscitation
- High concentration oxygen should be given through a reservoir mask.
- The wound should be sealed with an Asherman valve, if available. This is a device specifically designed to occlude an open pneumothorax. It incorporates a flutter valve which allows air to escape during expiration, preventing the development of a tension pneumothorax. (See Figure 16.1.)
- Traditionally, open pneumothoraces have been occluded by covering the wound and sealing it on three sides in order to allow air to escape. Although less effective, this may still be considered as an alternative (see Chapter 16) if an Asherman valve is not available.
- The hospital should be alerted and the child transferred urgently.

Flail chest

The elasticity of the child's chest wall reduces the incidence of flail chest. On the other hand, children who sustain these injuries are badly affected, because the increased mobility means that the underlying lung injury tends to be worse.

Signs
- The child will be hypoxic.
- Abnormal chest movement associated with rib crepitus may be observed.
- Flail segments may not be seen on initial examination since reflex splinting of the segment occurs.

Resuscitation
- High concentration oxygen should be given through a reservoir mask. Bag-and-mask ventilation should be considered.
- The hospital should be alerted and the child transferred urgently.
- Adequate pain relief in the form of intravenous analgesia (not Entonox, in the case of pneumothorax) should be given. Consider splinting the arm on the affected side to the chest wall for support.

Cardiac tamponade

Cardiac tamponade can occur after both penetrating or blunt injury. The blood that accumulates in the fibrous pericardial sac reduces the volume available for cardiac filling during diastole. As more blood accumulates, cardiac output is progressively reduced.

Signs
- The child will be in shock.
- There may be distended neck veins. This will not be apparent if significant hypovolaemia coexists.
- There may be muffled heart sounds (a difficult sign to detect in the pre-hospital environment).

Resuscitation
- High flow oxygen should be given through a reservoir mask.
- Emergency needle pericardiocentesis should be performed if suitably skilled personnel are available. Removal of a small volume of fluid from within the pericardium can dramatically increase cardiac output. Details of this are beyond the scope of this book.
- The hospital should be alerted and the child transferred urgently.

The following injuries cannot be accurately diagnosed on scene but will require specialist investigatory equipment to confirm them.

Pulmonary contusion

Children can absorb substantial amounts of kinetic energy through their chest wall with little or no initial signs of injury. The result of the energy transfer often manifests itself later, making careful monitoring essential.

Children have a high incidence of pulmonary contusion because of the mobility of the ribs. There may be no overlying fracture. This injury is usually the result of blunt trauma which ruptures pulmonary capillaries allowing blood to fill the alveoli and causing the child to become hypoxic.

Treatment consists of the administration of high flow oxygen, and artificial ventilation if necessary.

The hospital should be alerted and the child transferred urgently if this is suspected.

Tracheal and bronchial rupture

Frequently lethal, this presents as a pneumo- or haemopneumothorax, possibly with associated subcutaneous emphysema.

Immediate treatment consists of the administration of high concentration oxygen, drainage of any tension pneumothorax, and artificial ventilation if necessary.

The hospital should be alerted and the child transferred urgently if this is suspected.

Disruption of great vessels

This is usually rapidly fatal. A child with this injury who survives to get to hospital has a tear in a vessel which has tamponaded itself.

The patient may be shocked and peripheral pulses may be poorly palpable. Do not delay the transfer to gain intravenous access—use an intraosseous needle if access is necessary and difficult to obtain.

The hospital should be alerted if this is suspected and the child transferred urgently.

Ruptured diaphragm

This may occur following blunt abdominal trauma, and is more common on the left side. The child may be hypoxic due to pulmonary compression, and may have signs of hypovolaemia if intra-abdominal visceral injury has occurred.

The hospital should be alerted and the child transferred urgently.

Assessment: other injuries

Simple pneumothorax

A self-limiting leak of air occurs. This causes partial lung collapse. Signs of hypoxia are rarely apparent. Clinically, decreased chest wall movement, diminished breath sounds, and hyper-resonance may be found on the side of the pneumothorax.

The diagnosis will usually be made later, radiologically.

Those found on secondary survey

Attention must be given to life threatening injuries identified during the primary survey. During transportation the airway, breathing, circulation, and disability should be constantly reassessed and treated as necessary. Saturation and ECG monitoring should be initiated and baseline checks constantly observed and noted.

Once the child has been assessed and life threatening injuries excluded, the chest can be examined for less serious injuries.

Transportation

Any child with a significant chest injury who is being transported by helicopter should be transported at an altitude of less than 300 metres above the starting altitude. If this is not possible, ground transportation should be considered, or special precautions beyond the scope of this book may be required.

ABDOMINAL TRAUMA

Blunt trauma causes the majority of abdominal injuries in children. Most occur because of accidents on the roads, while a significant number happen during recreational activities. A high index of suspicion is necessary if some injuries are not to be missed.

The abdominal contents are very susceptible to injury in children for a number of reasons. The abdominal wall is thin and offers relatively little protection. The diaphragm is more horizontal than in adults, causing the liver and spleen to lie lower and more anteriorly. Furthermore, the ribs, being very elastic, offer less protection to these organs. Finally, the bladder is intra-abdominal, rather than pelvic, and is therefore more exposed. Respiratory compromise can complicate abdominal injury since diaphragmatic irritation or splinting may occur—reducing the use of the diaphragm during breathing.

115

Assessment

A precise history of the mechanism of injury will help in diagnosis. Rapid deceleration, such as experienced during road accidents, causes abdominal compression if seatbelts are incorrectly applied. The spleen and liver are at risk from such forces and the duodenum may develop a large haematoma or may even rupture. Direct blows, such as those caused by punching or impact with bicycle handlebars, injure underlying organs. Again, the liver and spleen, being relatively exposed, are at risk. Finally, straddling injuries can cause perineal injury and may rupture the urethra.

Primary survey

Initial assessment and management must be directed to the care of the airway, breathing, and circulation.

If shock is not amenable to fluid replacement following the primary survey and resuscitation, and no obvious site of haemorrhage exists, then intra-abdominal injury may be the cause of blood loss.

Crush injuries to the abdomen and pelvis   Both visceral damage and pelvic disruption can lead to life threatening blood loss. The child will present with hypovolaemic shock; this may remain resistant to treatment until either the pelvic disruption is stabilised or definitive surgical treatment has been provided in hospital.

Resuscitation

Initial treatment during the primary survey and resuscitation phase consists of oxygen administration and rapid fluid infusions to maintain the circulation during transportation to hospital. Splintage at this stage needs only to be in the form of packing the child to a spinal board. Urgent transfer to hospital is indicated.

Secondary survey

Gentle palpation should be carried out. This will reveal areas of tenderness and rigidity. Care should be taken not to hurt the child since continued cooperation is important during the repeated examinations which form an important part of management. The abdomen should be inspected for bruising, lacerations, and penetrating wounds. Major intra-abdominal injury can occur without obvious external signs, and visible bruising is therefore highly significant.

SUMMARY

Chest trauma

- Children have very compliant chest walls and may sustain significant chest injury without obvious external injury. The absence of external signs should not therefore be used to judge the severity of the injury.
- The first priorities are assessment and management of the airway with cervical spine immobilisation, breathing, circulation, and rapid assessment of conscious level using AVPU.
- All patients should receive high percentage oxygen through a reservoir mask.
- All children with chest injuries must be observed extremely carefully during transfer to hospital.
- Chest injuries can be life threatening but most can be managed successfully, using simple techniques

Abdominal trauma

- A history of the mechanism of injury will help the diagnosis of suspected abdominal injury.
- The first priorities are assessment and management of the airway with cervical spine immobilisation, breathing, circulation and rapid assessment of conscious level using AVPU.
- Tenderness or rigidity during palpation or signs of bruising or lacerations over the abdomen may identify underlying injury during the secondary survey.

Questions

1   List four serious injuries which may result from chest trauma.
2   What treatment is indicated for all serious chest injuries?
3   What assessment of the abdomen should be undertaken during the secondary survey following abdominal trauma?

13.3

Trauma to the extremities, burns, electrical injuries, and near drowning

OBJECTIVES
After reading this section you should be able to:

- State the potentially life threatening injuries associated with extremity trauma
- Describe the correct assessment and resuscitation of a child following extremity trauma
- Describe the correct assessment and resuscitation of a child with burns
- Identify the factors determining the effect of electrical injury
- Describe the correct assessment and resuscitation of a child following electrical injury
- Describe the correct assessment and resuscitation of a child following near drowning
- State the prognostic indicators following near drowning

INJURIES TO THE EXTREMITIES

It is uncommon for extremity trauma to be life threatening in the multiply injured child. It is crucial to recognise and treat associated life threatening injuries before assessing and managing the skeletal trauma. This section deals with problems from the perspective of multiple injury; the principles apply equally to individual injuries.

The differences between the mature and immature skeleton have a bearing on initial treatment and eventual outcome. Use of the principles usually applied to injuries of the mature skeleton will result in errors of both diagnosis and treatment. Unlike the adult skeleton, which is relatively static, the developing skeleton exhibits structural and functional changes, both physiological and biomechanical, which vary throughout growth. These result in different patterns of failure, healing response, and complications.

The two main differences are growth from the physis, and the structure of bone. Physeal injury or injury to an epiphyseal ossification centre may result in complete or partial arrest of growth; the latter results in progressive deformity. The relative proportions of lamellar and trabecular bone are constantly changing throughout life, which thus results in a change in fracture pattern as the child grows. Up to a certain point children's bones can spring back into shape. As deformation increases greenstick fractures and then complete fractures occur. The chances of fracture propagation are reduced and comminuted fractures are rare. It should be remembered that children's bones can absorb more force than adults and this may result in an underestimation of the degree of trauma to associated soft tissues.

In the growing child, fracture healing is more rapid and remodelling can occur.

Assessment

Unless extremity injury is life threatening, evaluation is carried out during the secondary survey. Single closed extremity injuries may produce enough blood loss to cause hypovolaemic shock but this is not usually life threatening. Multiple fractures can, however, cause severe shock. Pelvic fractures are relatively uncommon in children but the energy that would have fractured a pelvis in an adult may have been transmitted to vessels within the pelvis of a child, leading to disruption and haemorrhage. Closed fractures of the femur may cause loss of approximately 20% of the intravascular volume into the thigh and blood loss from open fractures can be significant. This blood loss begins at the time of the injury and it can be difficult to estimate the degree of pre-hospital loss. Careful assessment at the scene and continuous observation during transportation is therefore necessary.

Primary survey

All multiply injured children should be approached in the structured way discussed in Chapter 12. Relevant history should be sought from relatives and bystanders. Extremity deformity and perfusion prior to arrival at hospital are especially important and information concerning the mechanism of injury is helpful to hospital staff.

Potentially life threatening injuries include:

- Traumatic amputation of an extremity.
- Massive open long bone fractures.

These should be dealt with immediately, and take precedence over any other extremity injury.

Traumatic amputation Traumatic amputation of an extremity may be partial or complete. Paradoxically it is usually the former which presents the greatest initial threat to life. This is because completely transected vessels go into spasm while partially transected vessels do not. Blood loss can be severe and the pre-hospital care of these injuries is critical.

The airway should be cleared and breathing assessed as previously discussed. **Haemorrhage must be controlled**. If local pressure and elevation are not sufficient the application of a tourniquet should be considered. If this becomes necessary the tourniquet should be applied as distally as possible, and care should be taken to use a broad rather than a thin cuff. Orthopaedic pneumatic tourniquets are ideal but as these will not be available outside hospital, a sphygmomanometer cuff inflated to above arterial pressure may be used. The time of application should be recorded. Circulatory access should be obtained and shock treated. Urgent transfer to hospital is required.

Reimplantation techniques are available in specialist centres. The success rate is improving, particularly in children. Urgent referral and secondary transfer is necessary—the amputated part will only remain viable for 8 hours at room temperature, or for 18 hours if cooled. The amputated part should be cleaned, wrapped in a moist sterile towel, placed in a sterile, sealed plastic bag and transported, *in the same vehicle as the child*, in an insulated box filled with crushed ice and water. Care should be taken to avoid direct contact between the ice and tissue.

Massive open long bone fractures   The blood loss from any long bone fracture is significant; open fractures bleed more than closed ones since there is no tamponade effect from surrounding tissues. As a general rule an open fracture causes twice the blood loss of a corresponding closed fracture. Thus a single open femoral shaft fracture may result in 40% loss of circulating blood volume. This in itself is life threatening.

After airway and breathing have been assessed and treated, exsanguinating haemorrhage should be controlled both by the application of pressure at the fracture site and by correct splinting of the limb. The child should be transported to hospital. In transit, vascular access can be obtained and the child treated for shock. If intraosseous infusion is necessary, the needle should **not** be sited distal to the fracture.

Secondary survey

In a conscious child inspection is usually the most productive part of the examination. Causing pain or eliciting crepitus in an injured extremity will only increase anxiety, ultimately making the child more difficult to manage.

The extremities should be inspected for discoloration, bruising, swelling, deformity, lacerations, and evidence of open fractures.

Gentle palpation will establish any areas of tenderness. Capillary refill should be assessed, and pulses sought, although it is often impractical to assess distal lower limb pulses in the back of a moving ambulance.

The **viability of a limb** may be threatened by vascular injury, compartment syndrome, or by open fractures. These situations are discussed below.

Vascular injury   Assessment of the vascular status of the extremity is a key step in evaluating an injury. Vascular damage may be caused by traction (resulting in intimal damage or complete disruption), or by penetrating injuries from either a missile or the end of a fractured bone. Brisk bleeding from an open wound or a rapidly expanding mass are indicative of active bleeding. Complete tears are less likely to bleed for a prolonged period due to contraction of the vessel. It should be remembered that nerves usually pass in close proximity to vessels and are likely to have been damaged along with the vessel.

The presence of a pulse does not rule out a vascular injury. **A diminished pulse should not be attributed to spasm.** The characteristic signs are shown in Box 13.2.

Box 13.2   SIGNS OF VASCULAR INJURY

- Pale limb
- Impaired capillary return
- Decreased sensation
- Rapidly expanding haematoma
- Bruit (difficult to elicit pre-hospital)
- Abnormal pulses

If a vascular injury is suspected, the fracture should be aligned and splints checked to ensure that they are not restrictive. Vascular damage may not always be immediately apparent; constant reassessment is therefore important.

Compartment syndrome   If the interstitial pressure within a fascial compartment rises above capillary pressure, then local muscle ischaemia occurs. If this is unrecognised, it eventually results in Volkmann's ischaemic contracture.

Compartment syndrome usually develops over a period of hours and is most often associated with crush injuries. It may, however, occur following simple fractures. The characteristic signs are shown in Box 13.3.

Box 13.3 SIGNS OF COMPARTMENT SYNDROME

- Pain, accentuated by passively stretching the involved muscles
- Decreased sensation
- Swelling
- Weakness

Distal pulses only disappear when the intra-compartmental pressure rises above arterial pressure; by this time irreversible changes have usually occurred in the muscle bed. Initial treatment consists of releasing constricting bandages and splints.

The child should be transported to hospital without delay.

Open fractures Any wound within the vicinity of a fracture should be assumed to communicate with the fracture.

Open wounds are classified according to the degree of soft tissue damage, the amount of contamination, and the presence or absence of associated neurovascular damage. Initial treatment includes removal of gross contamination, and covering of the wound with a sterile dressing. Bleeding should be controlled by direct pressure.

Non-accidental injury This must always be considered if the history is not consistent with the injury pattern. It is discussed in detail in Appendix B.

Management

Life threatening problems identified during the primary survey in the multiply injured patient are managed first. Only then should attention be turned to the extremity injury. The specific management of complications such as vascular injury, compartment syndrome, traumatic amputation, and open wounds has been discussed earlier in this chapter.

This must not delay the patient's transfer to hospital.

Alignment

Severely angulated fractures should be aligned. Gentle traction should be applied to the limb to facilitate alignment, particularly when immobilising long bone fractures. Splints should extend one joint above and below the fracture site. Perfusion of the extremity, including pulses, skin colour, temperature, and neurological status must be assessed before and after the fracture is aligned.

When aligning a fracture, analgesia is usually necessary. Entonox or intravenous opiates should be used. In femoral fractures, femoral nerve block is very effective but is often impractical in the pre-hospital setting.

Immobilisation

Fractures (or suspected fractures) should be immobilised to control pain and prevent further injury. Splintage is a most effective way of controlling pain and subsequent doses of analgesia may be reduced. If pain increases after immobilisation, then an ischaemic injury and/or compartment syndrome must be excluded. Emergency splinting techniques for various injured extremities are described below.

Upper limb • **Hand**
  This should be elevated and kept comfortable.

  • **Forearm and wrist**
  Splinted flat on padded pillows or splints.

121

- **Elbow**
  Immobilised in a flexed position with a sling which may be strapped to the body.

- **Arm**
  Immobilised by a sling, which can be augmented with splints for unstable fractures. Circumferential bandages should be avoided as they may be the cause of constriction, particularly when swelling occurs.

- **Shoulder**
  Immobilised by a sling.

Lower limb
- **Femur**
  Femoral fractures should be treated in traction splints. Ipsilateral femoral and tibial fractures can be immobilised in the same splint. Excess traction may cause perineal injury and neurovascular problems, and should be avoided. Traction splintage should not be applied to patients with pelvic fractures.

- **Tibia and ankle**
  Tibial and ankle fractures should be aligned and immobilised in padded box splints. Foot perfusion should be assessed before and after application of the splint.

BURNS

Epidemiology

Each year some 20 000 burned and 30 000 scalded children attend Accident and Emergency departments. Of these, 5000–6000 require hospital admission. In England and Wales in 1997, 56 children died from burns. Of those burned, 70% are pre-school children, the commonest age being between 1 and 2 years. Scalds occur mostly in the under-4s. Boys are more likely to suffer burns and serious scalds.

Most fatal burns occur in house fires and smoke inhalation is the usual cause of death. The number of deaths from burns has decreased because of a combination of factors. The move away from open fires, safer fireguards, and more stringent low flammability requirements for night clothes have all played their parts. Non-fatal burns often involve clothing and are often associated with flammable liquids. They show no sign of decreasing in number.

Scalds are usually caused by hot drinks, but bath water and cooking oil scalds are not uncommon. The improvement in survival following scalding (which followed improvements in treatment) has reached a plateau.

There is a strong link between burns to children and low socioeconomic status. Family stress, poor housing conditions, and overcrowding are implicated in this.

Pathophysiology

Two main factors determine the severity of burns and scalds—these are the temperature and the duration of contact. The time taken for cellular destruction to occur decreases exponentially with temperature. At 44 °C contact would have to be maintained for 6 hours, at 54 °C for 30 seconds, and at 70 °C epidermal injury happens within a second.

This relationship underlies the different patterns of injury seen with different types of burn. Scalds generally involve water at below boiling point and contact for less than 4 seconds. Scalds that occur with liquids at a higher temperature (such as hot fat), or in children incapable of minimising the contact time (such as young infants and the

122

handicapped) tend to result in more serious injuries. Flame burns can involve high temperatures and prolonged contact and consequently produce the most serious injuries of all. It must be re-emphasised that the most common cause of death within the first hour following burn injuries is smoke inhalation. Thus, as with other types of injury, attention to airway and breathing is of prime importance.

Primary survey and resuscitation

When faced with a seriously burned child it is easy to focus on the immediate problems of the burn, and forget the possibility of other injuries. The approach to the burned child should be the systematic assessment of the ABCs as advocated in the initial assessment chapter. Before approaching the child, the scene of the incident must be assessed for safety and attendance of the fire service requested if required.

Airway and cervical spine

The airway may be compromised either because of inhalational injury, or because of severe burns to the face. The latter are usually obvious whereas the former may only be indicated more subtly. The indicators of inhalational injury are shown in Box 13.4.

> **Box 13.4 INDICATIONS OF INHALATIONAL INJURY**
>
> - History of exposure to smoke in a confined space
> - Deposits around the mouth and nose
> - Carbonaceous sputum

Since oedema occurs following thermal injury, the airway can deteriorate rapidly. Thus even suspicion of airway compromise, or the discovery of injuries which might be expected to cause problems with the airway at a later stage, should lead to immediate consideration of endotracheal intubation. This procedure increases in difficulty as oedema progresses, and it is important to perform it as soon as possible. All but the most experienced should seek expert help urgently, unless apnoea requires immediate intervention. This usually means immediate evacuation to hospital.

If there is any suspicion of cervical spine injury, or if the history is unobtainable, appropriate precautions should be taken until such injury is excluded.

Breathing

Once the airway has been secured, the adequacy of breathing should be assessed. Signs which should arouse suspicion of inadequacy include: abnormal respiratory rate, abnormal chest movements, and cyanosis (a late sign). Circumferential burns to the chest may cause breathing difficulty by mechanically restricting chest movement.

All children who have suffered burns should be given high concentration oxygen. If there are signs of breathing problems then ventilation should be considered.

Circulation

In the first few hours following injury signs of hypovolaemic shock are rarely attributable to burns. Therefore any such signs should raise the suspicion of bleeding from elsewhere, and the source should be actively sought. Vascular access should be obtained in unburned areas, but eschar can be perforated if necessary. Remember that the intraosseous route can be used, although it is not preferred.

Disability

Reduced conscious level following burns may be due to hypoxia (following smoke inhalation), head injury, or hypovolaemia. It is essential that a quick AVPU assessment is made during the primary survey since this provides a baseline for later observations.

123

Exposure

Exposure should be brief. Burned children lose heat especially rapidly, and must be covered with blankets when not being examined.

Assessing the burn

The severity of a burn depends on its relative surface area and depth. Burns to particular areas may require special care.

Surface area   The surface area is usually estimated using burns charts. It is particularly important to use a paediatric chart when assessing burn size in children, since the relative surface areas of the head and limbs change with age. This variation is illustrated in the body surface area chart (Figure 2.3) found in Chapter 2 of this manual.

Another useful method of estimating relative surface area relies on the fact that the patient's palm and adducted fingers cover an area of approximately 1% of the body surface. This method can be used when charts are not immediately available and may therefore be more practical in the pre-hospital setting.

Note that the "Rule of Nines" cannot be applied to a child who is less than 14 years old.

Depth   Burns are classified as being superficial, partial thickness or full thickness. The first causes injury only to the epidermis and clinically the skin appears red with no blister formation. Partial thickness burns cause some damage to the dermis; blistering is usually seen and the skin is pink or mottled. Deeper (full thickness) burns damage both the epidermis and dermis, and may cause injury to deeper structures as well. The skin looks white or charred, and is painless and leathery to touch.

Special areas   Burns to the face and mouth have already been dealt with above. Burns involving the hand can cause severe functional loss if scarring occurs. Perineal burns are prone to infection and present particularly difficult management problems.

Initial burn care

Analgesia

Most burned children will be in severe pain, and this should be dealt with urgently. Some older children may manage to use Entonox, but most will not. Any child with burns that are anything other than minor should be given *intravenous* morphine at a dose of 0.1 mg/kg as soon as possible. There is no place for administration of intramuscular analgesia in severe burns since absorption is unreliable.

Wound care

Infection is a significant cause of mortality and morbidity in burns victims, and wound care should start as early as possible to reduce this risk. Furthermore, appropriate wound care will reduce the pain associated with air passing over burned areas.

Burns should be covered with cling film or sterile towels, and unnecessary re-examination should be avoided. Blisters should be left intact. Although cold compresses and irrigation with cold water may reduce pain, it should be remembered that burned children lose heat rapidly. These treatments should only be used for 10 minutes or less, and only in patients with partial thickness burns totalling less than 10%. **Children should *never* be transported with cold soaks in place.**

Secondary survey

As well as being burned, children may suffer the effects of blast, may be injured by falling objects, and may fall while trying to escape from the fire. Thus other injuries are not uncommon and a head-to-toe secondary survey should be carried out. Any injuries discovered, including the burn, should be treated in order of priority.

ELECTRICAL INJURIES

Epidemiology

Children account for 33% of all victims of electrical injuries; approximately 20% of reported electrical injuries are fatal. Over 90% result from accidents involving generated electricity.

Pathophysiology

The following factors determine the effects of an electric shock.

Current Alternating current (AC) produces cardiac arrest at lower voltage than does direct current (DC). Whether electrocution is with AC or DC, the risk of cardiac arrest is greater with increasing size and duration of current passing through the heart; the current will be greater with low resistance and high voltage.

Lightning acts as a massive DC countershock which depolarises the myocardium and may lead to immediate asystole and death.

As current increases the following may be seen:

- **Above 10 mA**: tetanic contractions of muscles may make it impossible for the child to let go of the electrical source.
- **50 mA**: tetanic contraction of the diaphragm and intercostal muscles leads to respiratory arrest which continues until the current is disconnected. If hypoxia is prolonged, secondary cardiac arrest will occur.
- **Over 100 mA to several amps**: primary cardiac arrest may be induced (defibrillators used in resuscitation deliver around 10 A).
- **50 A to hundreds of amps**: massive shocks cause prolonged respiratory and cardiac arrest, and more severe burns.

Resistance The resistance of tissues determines the path that the current follows. In general, this is the path of least resistance from the entry point on the victim to ground. Thus current preferentially flows down nerves and blood vessels rather than through muscles, skin, tendon, fat or bone. Electrocution of tissues with high resistance will generate most heat, and tissues tolerate this to varying degrees. Overall nerves, blood vessels, skin and muscle sustain most injury.

Water reduces skin resistance and thereby increases the current delivered to the body.

Voltage High voltage ("tension") sources such as overhead electric power lines or lightning involve a higher current, and consequently cause more tissue damage than lower voltage sources.

Primary survey

Prior to commencing treatment it is essential that the area is safe to approach and the child is disconnected from the electric source.

Primary survey is undertaken following the ABC principles, as with all trauma casualties.

Resuscitation

The airway may be compromised by facial burns, and early management of such problems is essential. If the child is unconscious, the neck should be assumed to be unstable and must be protected until injury is excluded. Other life threatening injuries may occur during secondary trauma and must be treated appropriately.

Secondary survey

Virtually any injury can occur. In particular, associated injuries can arise from being thrown from the source. Burns are common, and happen either because of the direct effects of the current (exit burns are often more severe than entry burns), or secondary to the ignition of clothing. The powerful tetanic contraction caused by the shock can cause fractures or muscle tearing.

NEAR DROWNING

Drowning is defined as death from asphyxia associated with submersion in a fluid. Near drowning is said to have occurred if there is any recovery (however transient) following a submersion incident.

Epidemiology

The incidence of near drowning is unknown, but drowning is the third commonest cause of accidental death in children in the UK (after road accidents and burns). In England and Wales the annual incidence of submersion accidents in under-15-year-olds is 1.5 per 100 000 and the mortality in this age group is 0.7 per 100 000. The highest incidence (3.6 per 100 000) occurs in boys under 5 years old. Children most commonly die in private swimming pools, garden ponds, and inland waterways.

Pathophysiology

When a child is first submerged breath holding occurs and the heart rate slows because of the diving reflex. As apnoea continues hypoxia causes tachycardia, a rise in the blood pressure and acidosis. Between 20 seconds and $2\frac{1}{2}$ minutes later a break point is reached, and breathing occurs. Fluid is inhaled and on touching the glottis causes immediate laryngeal spasm. Secondary apnoea eventually gives way to involuntary respiratory movements, and water, weeds, and debris enter the lungs. Bradycardia and arrhythmias follow, heralding cardiac arrest and death.

Children who survive because of interruption of this chain of events not only require therapy for near drowning, but also assessment and treatment of concomitant hypothermia, electrolyte imbalance, and injury (particularly spinal).

Primary survey and resuscitation

The neck must be presumed to be injured, and the cervical spine should be immobilised until such injury is excluded. A history of diving is especially significant in this regard.

Following a significant near drowning episode the stomach is usually full of swallowed water. The risk of aspiration is therefore increased and tracheal intubation should therefore be considered.

A core temperature reading must be obtained as soon as possible. Hypothermia is common following near drowning, and adversely affects resuscitation attempts unless treated. Not only are arrhythmias more common, but some, such as ventricular fibrillation, may be refractory at temperatures below 30 °C. Resuscitation should not be discontinued until core temperature is at least 32 °C.

Rewarming

External rewarming is usually sufficient if the core temperature is above 32 °C. Active core rewarming should be added in patients with a core temperature of less than 32 °C, but beware "rewarming shock" which may result from hypovolaemia becoming apparent during peripheral vasodilatation. Core rewarming outside hospital is likely to be limited to warm intravenous fluids. Alternatively, a wide range of core rewarming methods is available in hospital and therefore transport to hospital should not be delayed.

External and internal rewarming methods are:

External rewarming

1   Remove cold, wet clothing. Apply warm blankets.
2   Infrared radiant lamp.
3   Heating blanket.

Core rewarming available in hospital

1   Warm intravenous fluids to 37 °C.
2   Warm ventilator gases to 42 °C.
3   Gastric or bladder lavage with normal saline at 42 °C.
4   Peritoneal lavage with potassium free dialysate at 42 °C.
5   Pleural or pericardial lavage.
6   Extracorporeal blood rewarming.

ECG monitoring and constant monitoring of vital signs should be undertaken in transit.

Secondary survey

During the secondary survey, the child should be carefully examined from head to toe in a warm, dry environment. Any injury may have occurred during the incident that preceded submersion; spinal injuries are particularly common.

Prognostic indicators

Immersion time   Most children who do not recover have been submerged for more than 3–8 minutes. Details of the rescue are therefore vital.

Time to first gasp   If this occurs between 1 and 3 minutes after the start of basic cardiopulmonary support the prognosis is good. If there has been no gasp after 40 minutes of full CPR there is little or no chance of survival unless the child's respiration has been depressed (for example by hypothermia or alcohol).

Rectal temperature   If this is less than 33 °C on arrival the chances of survival are increased since rapid cooling protects vital organs. Children cool quickly because of their large surface area/volume ratio.

Persisting coma   This indicates a bad prognosis.

Type of water   Whether the water was salt or fresh has no bearing on the prognosis.

Outcome

Seventy per cent of children survive near drowning when basic life support is provided at the waterside. Only 40% survive without early basic life support even if full advanced CPR is given in hospital.

Of those who do survive having required full CPR in hospital, around 70% will make a complete recovery and 25% will have a mild neurological deficit. The remainder will be severely disabled or remain in a persisting vegetative state.

SUMMARY

Trauma to the extremities

- Extremity trauma is rarely life threatening per se, unless exsanguinating haemorrhage ensues. Multiple fractures can cause significant blood loss.
- The first priority is assessment of the airway, breathing, and circulation.
- Full assessment of the extremities takes place during the secondary survey. Limb threatening injuries should be identified at this stage and management begun.

Burns

- The first priority is assessment of the airway, breathing, and circulation.
- An assessment should be made of the area, depth, and site of the burn.
- Children should never be transported with cold soaks in place.

Electrical injuries

- The factors determining the outcome of electric shock are current, resistance and voltage.
- Assessment and safe approach to the scene are essential.

Near drowning

- There is a high incidence of associated cervical spine injury, especially during diving accidents.
- Other associated injuries may arise during the incident leading to submersion.
- Hypothermia should be considered and treated where possible—resuscitation attempts must not be abandoned until the patient reaches hospital and the core temperature is at least 32 °C.

Questions

1 List two types of life threatening extremity injury.
2 In what ways are children's bones different from adult bones?
3 What is the primary concern when attending a child with an electrical injury?
4 List two good prognostic factors in a near drowned child.

14

Procedures: airway and breathing

OBJECTIVES

After reading this chapter you should understand the correct methods of performing the following procedures:

- Oropharyngeal airway insertion
    small child
    older child
- Nasopharyngeal airway insertion
- Orotracheal intubation
    infant/small child
    older child
- Ventilation without intubation
    mouth-to-mask ventilation
    bag-and-mask ventilation

OROPHARYNGEAL AIRWAY INSERTION

If the gag reflex is present, it may be best to avoid the use of an oropharyngeal tube or other artificial airway, since they may cause choking, laryngospasm or vomiting (see Chapter 7).

Small child

1 Select an appropriate size of Guedel airway (see Chapter 7).
2 Open the airway using the chin lift, taking care not to move the neck if trauma has occurred.
3 Use a tongue depressor or a laryngoscope blade to aid insertion of the airway "the right way up" (Figure 14.1).
4 Re-check the airway patency.
5 If necessary, consider a different size from the original estimate.
6 Finally, provide oxygen and consider ventilation by pocket mask or bag and mask.

Older child

1 Select an appropriate size of Guedel airway (see Chapter 7).
2 Open the airway using the chin lift, taking care not to move the neck if trauma has occurred.

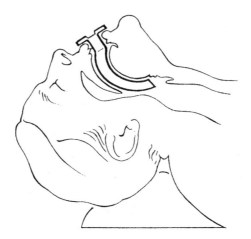

Figure 14.1. Orotracheal airway *in situ*

3 Insert the airway concave surface upwards until the tip reaches the soft palate.
4 Rotate it through 180° (convex side upwards) and slide it back over the tongue.
5 Re-check the airway patency.
6 If necessary, consider a different size from the original estimate.
7 Finally provide oxygen and consider ventilation by pocket mask or bag and mask.

NASOPHARYNGEAL AIRWAY INSERTION

Assess for any contraindications such as a possible base of skull fracture.

1 Select an appropriate size (length and diameter) (see Chapter 7).
2 Lubricate the airway with a water-soluble lubricant, and insert a large safety pin through the flange.
3 Insert the tip into the nostril and direct it posteriorly along the floor of the nose (rather than upwards) (Figure 14.2).

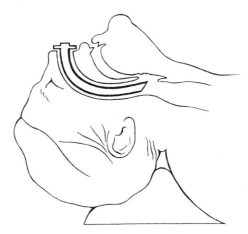

Figure 14.2. Nasopharyngeal airway *in situ*

4 Gently pass the airway past the turbinates with a slight rotating motion. As the tip advances into the pharynx, there should be a palpable "give".
5 Continue until the flange and safety pin rest on the nostril.
6 If there is difficulty inserting the airway, consider using the other nostril or a smaller size from the original estimate.
7 Re-check the airway patency.
8 Finally, provide oxygen and consider ventilation by pocket mask or bag and mask.

OROTRACHEAL INTUBATION

Infant or small child

1 Ensure that adequate ventilation and oxygenation by face mask are in progress.
2 Select an appropriate laryngoscope, and check the brightness of the light.
3 Select an appropriate tube size, but prepare a range of sizes, including the size above and below the best estimate (see Chapter 7).
4 Ensure manual immobilisation of the neck by an assistant if cervical spine injury is possible. Because of the relatively large occiput, it may be helpful to place a folded sheet or towel under the baby's back and neck to allow correct positioning of the head.
5 Hold the laryngoscope in the left hand, and insert it into the right hand side of the mouth, displacing the tongue to the left. In the infant, it is sometimes useful to hold the laryngoscope with the left thumb and index and middle fingers, leaving the little finger free to stretch down to press on the larynx to improve the view of the cords. This is particularly useful when working single-handed.
6 In the "flat" baby being intubated by a relatively inexperienced person, it is often easiest to place the laryngoscope blade well beyond the epiglottis. The laryngoscope blade is placed down the right hand side of the tongue into the proximal oesophagus. With a careful lifting movement, the tissues are gently tented up to "seek the midline". The blade is then slowly withdrawn until the cords come into view. In some situations, it may be better to stay proximal to the epiglottis to minimise the risk of causing laryngospasm. This decision must be based on clinical judgement.
7 Insert the endotracheal tube into the trachea, concentrating on how far the tip is being placed below the cords. The tip should lie 2–4 cm below the cords depending on age. Be aware that flexion or extension of the neck may cause migration downwards or upwards, respectively.
8 Check the placement of the tube by inspecting the chest for movement and auscultating the chest (including the axillae) and epigastrium.
9 If endotracheal intubation is not achieved in 30 seconds, discontinue the attempt, ventilate and oxygenate by mask, and try again.
10 Observe the chest wall movement. Monitor the oxygen saturation continuously. Tubes dislodge and block very easily.
11 Ensure that the tube is secured firmly in place and that no complications have occurred (see below).

Older child

1 Ensure that adequate ventilation and oxygenation by face mask are in progress.
2 Select an appropriate laryngoscope, and check the brightness of the light.
3 Select an appropriate tube size, but prepare a range of sizes, including the size above and below the best estimate (see Chapter 7).
4 Ensure manual immobilisation of the neck by an assistant if cervical spine injury is possible.
5 Hold the laryngoscope in the left hand, and insert it into the right hand side of the mouth, displacing the tongue to the left.
6 Visualise the epiglottis, and place the tip of the laryngoscope in the vallecula.
7 Gently but firmly lift the handle "towards the ceiling on the far side of the room", being careful not to lever on the teeth (see Figure 14.3).
8 Insert the endotracheal tube into the trachea, concentrating on how far the tip is being placed below the cords. The tip should lie 2–4 cm below the cords depending on age. If the tube has a "vocal cord level" marker, place this at the cords. Be aware that flexion or extension of the neck may cause migration downwards or upwards, respectively.

133

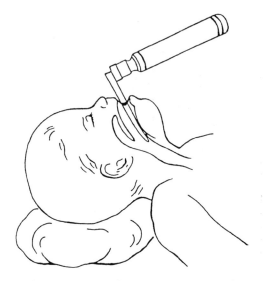

Figure 14.3. Intubation laryngoscope direction

9 In the adolescent, inflate the cuff to provide an adequate seal. In the pre-pubertal child do not use a cuffed tube.
10 Check the placement of the tube by inspecting the chest for movement and auscultating the chest (including the axillae) and epigastrium.
11 If endotracheal intubation is not achieved in 30 seconds, discontinue the attempt, ventilate and oxygenate by mask, and try again.
12 Observe the chest wall movement and monitor oxygen saturation continuously.
13 Ensure the tube is secured firmly in place and that no complications have occurred (see below).

Complications of endotracheal intubation
These include:

● Oesophageal intubation (causing severe hypoxia if not immediately recognised).
● Endobronchial intubation, resulting in lung collapse and risk of pneumothorax.
● Severe hypoxia from a prolonged attempt to intubate.
● Induction of vomiting and risk of aspiration.
● Airway injury from the laryngoscope, tube or stylet (including direct trauma to the vocal cords, as well as chipping or loosening of the teeth).
● Neck strain by overextension, or exacerbation of a cervical spine injury with risk of neurological deterioration.

VENTILATION WITHOUT INTUBATION

Mouth-to-mask ventilation

1 Apply the mask to the face, using a jaw thrust grip, with the thumbs holding the mask. If using a shaped mask, it should be the right way up in children (Figure 14.4), or upside down in infants.
2 Ensure an adequate seal.
3 Blow into the mouth port, observing the resulting chest movement.
4 Ventilate at 15–30 breaths/minute depending on the age of the child.
5 Attach oxygen to the face mask if possible.

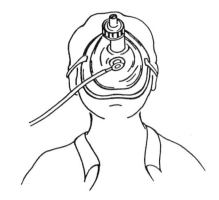

Figure 14.4. Mouth-to-mask ventilation

Bag-and-mask ventilation

1 Apply the mask to the face, using a jaw thrust grip, with a thumb holding the mask (see Figure 14.5).
2 Ensure an adequate seal.
3 Squeeze the bag observing the resulting chest movement.
4 Ventilate at 15–30 breaths/minute depending on the age of the child.

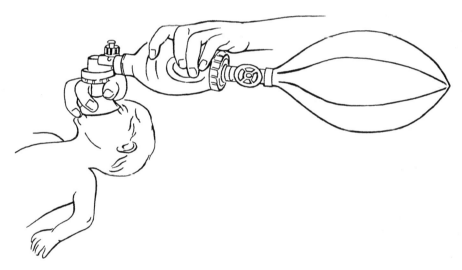

Figure 14.5. Bag-and-mask ventilation

If a two-person technique is used, one rescuer maintains the mask seal with both hands, while the second person squeezes the self-inflating bag. A two-person technique is preferable, but often impractical outside hospital because of the limited number of personnel.

15

Procedures: circulation

OBJECTIVES

After reading this chapter you should understand the correct methods of performing the following procedures:

- Vascular access
    - upper and lower extremity veins
    - scalp veins
- Intraosseous infusion
- Defibrillation

VASCULAR ACCESS

Access to the circulation is a crucial step in delivering Advanced Paediatric Life Support. Many access routes are possible; the one chosen will reflect both clinical need and the skills of the operator.

The search for a vein can usually be performed while the child is being transported to hospital. Once a vein (or bony area in the case of intraosseous infusion) is identified, the cannula and site can be prepared and the vehicle stopped briefly to insert the needle. Securing the cannula and fluid and drug administration can again be done in transit.

Peripheral venous access

Try to avoid leaving a tourniquet on a child longer than is necessary. Tourniquets are uncomfortable and frightening. It is better if possible to ask a parent or carer to squeeze the limb with their hand rather than use a tourniquet. This will also assist in keeping the limb immobilised for needle insertion.

Veins on the dorsum of the hand, the antecubital fossa, and the saphenous vein at the ankle can be used for cannulation. Standard percutaneous techniques should be employed, if possible. Always check a glucose level on any blood that flashes back on insertion.

Equipment

- Skin cleansing swabs.
- Suitable sized cannula.
- Three-way tap with short extension set, flushed with 0.9% saline.
- Syringe and 0.9% saline.
- Adhesive tape.

Procedure

1 Locate a vein.
2 Restrain the child.
3 Ask someone to squeeze the limb proximally or apply a tourniquet.
4 Clean the skin.
5 Stop the vehicle.
6 Insert the cannula and attach the three-way tap with flushed line.
7 Release the pressure on the limb (hand or tourniquet).
8 Recommence the journey.
9 Secure the cannula with tape.
10 Flush the cannula via the three-way tap with 2–5 ml of saline and ensure there is no swelling around the site.
11 Commence drug administration or bolus fluid administration as required.

Scalp veins

The frontal superficial temporal posterior, auricular, supraorbital, and posterior facial veins can be used. Although used commonly in the past, intraosseous infusion is often considered preferable nowadays because of its ease and stability.

Equipment

- Skin cleansing swabs.
- Paediatric cannula or butterfly needle.
- Syringe flushed with 0.9% saline. Three-way tap with extension set flushed with 0.9% saline.
- Short piece of tubing or bandage.
- Adhesive tape for securing.

Procedure: butterfly needle

1 Restrain the child.
2 Shave the appropriate area of the scalp, having located a vein.
3 Clean the skin.
4 Have an assistant distend the vein by holding a taut piece of tubing or bandaging perpendicular to it, proximal to the site of puncture.
5 Fill the syringe with 0.9% saline and flush the butterfly set.
6 Stop the vehicle.
7 Insert the needle under the skin.
8 Disconnect the syringe and leave the end of the tubing open.
9 Enter the vein. Blood will flow back through the tubing.
10 Infuse a small quantity of fluid to see that the cannula is properly placed. Attach the three-way tap and then tape into position.
11 Recommence the journey.

Procedure: paediatric cannula

This is the same as for peripheral cannulation except that it is not possible to squeeze the limb proximally to distend the vein. It is, however, possible to occlude the vein as in step 4 of the butterfly needle method.

Whichever method is used, if the skin around the infusion area blanches on flushing with saline, or the blood is pulsatile, the cannula/needle should be removed. It is likely to be in an artery.

Intraosseous transfusion

The technique of intraosseous transfusion is not new. It was used in the 1930s as a quick method of gaining vascular access (the only alternatives were to use a reusable, resharpened metal needle or perform a venous cutdown). Because it is important to achieve vascular access quickly in many life threatening situations, intraosseous infusion is again being recommended. Specially designed needles make this quick and easy. It is indicated if other attempts at venous access fail, or if they will take longer than 2 minutes to carry out.

Equipment

- Alcohol swabs.
- Size 16 G needle with trochar (at least 1.5 cm in length).
- 5 ml syringe.
- Three-way tap with short extension set, flushed with 0.9% saline.
- Orange "box" splint.
- 20 ml syringe, or 50 ml syringe as appropriate.
- Infusion fluid.

Procedure

1 Identify the infusion site. Fractured bones should be avoided, as should limbs with fractures proximal to possible sites. The landmarks for the upper tibial and lower femoral sites are shown in Table 15.1, and the former approach is illustrated in Figure 15.1.

Table 15.1. Surface anatomy for intraosseous infusions

Tibial	Femoral
Anterior surface, 2–3 cm below the tibial tuberosity	Anterolateral surface, 3 cm above the lateral condyle

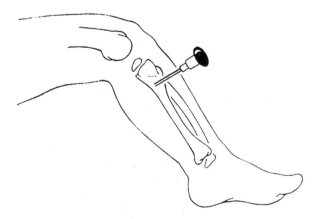

Figure 15.1. Tibial technique for intraosseous infusion

2 Clean the site.
3 Stop the vehicle.
4 Insert the needle at 90° to the skin.
5 Continue to advance the needle using a twisting motion until a "give" is felt as the cortex is penetrated.
6 Attach the 5 ml syringe and aspirate bone marrow to check position.
7 Recommence journey.
8 Check glucose level on bone marrow aspirated.

138

9 Attach a three-way tap.

10 Push in fluid boluses as required. Gravity dependent intravenous fluid administration sets will not flow via this route.

11 Immobilise leg in orange box splint (or similar) for easy identification.

DEFIBRILLATION

In order to achieve the optimum outcome defibrillation must be performed quickly and efficiently. This requires:

- Correct paddle position.
- Correct paddle placement.
- Good paddle contact.
- Correct energy selection.

Many defibrillators are available. Pre-hospital Paediatric Life Support providers should make sure they are familiar with those they may have to use. Automatic/semi-automatic defibrillators cannot be used in children because of the different energy requirements of children compared to adults.

Correct paddle selection

Most defibrillators are supplied with adult paddles attached (13 cm diameter, or equivalent area); 4.5 cm diameter paddles are suitable for use in infants, and 8 cm diameter should be used for small children (if available).

Correct paddle placement

The usual placement is anterolateral. One paddle is put over the apex in the mid-axillary line, and the other is placed just to the right of the sternum, immediately below the clavicle (Figure 15.2).

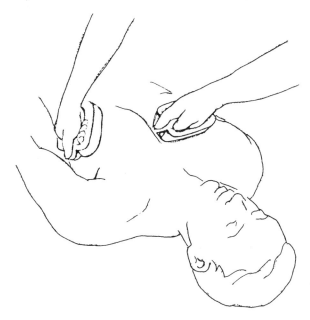

Figure 15.2. Standard anterior paddle placement

If the anteroposterior placement is used, one paddle is placed just to the left side of the lower part of the sternum, and the other just below the tip of the left scapula (Figure 15.3).

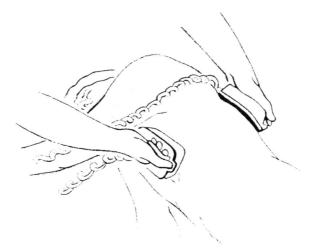

Figure 15.3. Anteroposterior paddle placement

Good paddle contact

Gel pads should always be used. Firm pressure should be applied to the paddles.

Correct energy selection

The recommended levels are shown in Chapter 8.

Safety

A defibrillator delivers enough current to *cause* cardiac arrest. The user must ensure that other rescuers are not in either direct or indirect (pools of water etc) physical contact with the patient (or the trolley) at the moment the shock is delivered. The defibrillator should only be charged when the paddles are correctly positioned on the child's chest.

Procedure

> **Basic life support should be interrupted for the shortest possible time (4–9 below)**

1. Apply gel pads or electrode gel.
2. Select the correct paddles.
3. Select the energy required.
4. Place the electrodes onto the pads of gel, and apply firm pressure.
5. Press the charge button.
6. Wait until the defibrillator is charged.
7. Shout "Stand back!"
8. Check that all other rescuers are clear.
9. Deliver the shock.
10. Reassess the rhythm.

CHAPTER

16

Procedures: trauma

> **OBJECTIVES**
>
> After reading this chapter you should understand the correct methods of performing the following procedures:
>
> - Application of three-way seal/Asherman valve
> - Needle thoracocentesis
> - Cervical collar application
> - Application of padding and tape
> - Log-rolling
> - Spinal board application
> - Rapid extrication
> - Crash helmet removal
> - Femoral nerve block

SEALING OPEN CHEST WOUNDS

An open sucking chest wound can be potentially devastating to trauma patients. They are dealt with as part of the "B" of the primary survey, after ensuring the patient's airway is patent. The aim of treatment is to seal the wound, allowing excess air pressure within the chest out but preventing air being drawn back into the thorax.

Asherman valve

Recently the Asherman valve (Figure 16.1) has become a popular method of sealing these wounds. This is a round adhesive disc with a flutter type valve attached. It can be used to seal punctures and the more common tear type wound.

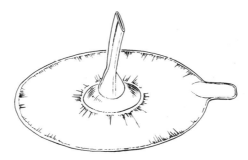

Figure 16.1. Asherman valve

Three-way seal

Traditionally sucking chest wounds are sealed using a square of plastic sealed on three sides. Recently doubt has been cast upon the efficiency of this method. If no

141

Asherman valve is available then this method may improve the situation. Remember, whichever method you choose, it is vital you constantly reassess the patient's condition; you may have made things worse!

CHEST DECOMPRESSION

Needle thoracocentesis

This procedure can be life saving and can be performed quickly with minimum equipment. It is indicated for suspected tension pneumothorax.

Minimum equipment

1   Alcohol swabs.
2   Large over-the-needle intravenous cannula (16 G and larger).
3   20 ml syringe.
4   Tape.

Procedure

1   Identify the second intercostal space in the mid-clavicular line on the side of the pneumothorax (the *opposite* side to the direction of tracheal deviation).
2   Swab the chest wall with surgical prep solution or an alcohol swab.
3   Attach the syringe to the cannula.
4   Insert the cannula into the chest wall, just above the rib below, aspirating all the time (Figure 16.2).

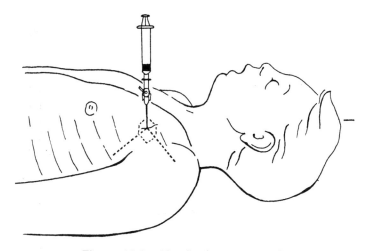

Figure 16.2.   Needle thoracocentesis

5   If air is aspirated, remove the needle, leaving the plastic cannula in place.
6   Tape the cannula in place and consider putting in a chest drain before transfer.

> If needle thoracocentesis is attempted, and the patient does not have a tension pneumothorax, the chance of causing a pneumothorax is 10–20%. Patients who have had this procedure must have a chest radiograph and will require chest drainage if ventilated

> Needle thoracocentesis must be followed by chest drain placement in hospital

SPINAL CARE

Cervical spine immobilisation

Although the majority of trauma patients will probably not sustain significant cervical trauma, it is impossible to exclude this on the scene. It is therefore advisable to treat all children with serious trauma as though they have a cervical spine injury and immobilise them accordingly. It is only when adequate investigations have been carried out and, if necessary, neurological and orthopaedic consultation completed, that the decision to remove cervical spine protection can be taken.

> There will never be adequate resources at the scene to allow cervical spine injury to be excluded

Manual in-line stabilisation, as shown in Figure 16.3, should be maintained until a hard collar has been applied and an appropriate head immobilisation device is fitted. The child's head may have to be moved to achieve a neutral in-line position as this is preferable to transporting the child with the head in an angulated position. Moving the head to an in-line position will also enable a cervical collar to be applied. Any attempt to move the child's head into an in-line position should be stopped if:

- **There is resistance to movement.**
- **Movement causes pain.**
- **Any increased neurological deficit is observed.**

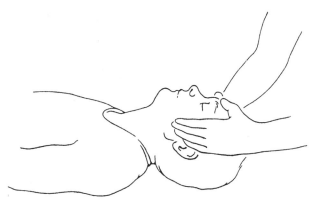

Figure 16.3. In-line cervical stabilisation

Remember when manually immobilising the head, not to cover the patient's ears with your hands. Covering the ears reduces communication with the child and may frighten them.

It must be remembered that, particularly under the age of 12 months, children have large occiputs. This means the neck has a tendency to flex. A small pad under the shoulders will help to maintain the head in the neutral position.

If in-line immobilisation is not possible, manual immobilisation will have to be maintained in the position found and the head immobilised using improvised equipment such as towels and blankets.

Cervical collar application and head immobilisation techniques are described below and it is necessary to use both to achieve cervical spine control.

Application of a cervical collar

Minimum equipment

1 Measuring device (if appropriate).
2 Range of paediatric hard collars.

> The key to successful, effective collar application lies in selecting the correct size

> Cervical collars alone will not fully immobilise the head

Procedure

1 Ensure that manual in line cervical stabilisation is maintained by a second person throughout.
2 Correctly size the collar.
3 Fully unfold and assemble the collar.
4 Taking care not to cause movement, pass the flat part of the collar behind the neck.
5 Fold the shaped part of the collar round and place it under the casualty's chin.
6 Fold the flat part of the collar with its integral joining device (usually Velcro tape) around until it meets the shaped part.
7 Reassess the fit of the collar.
8 If the fit is wrong, slip the flat part of the collar out from behind the neck, taking care not to cause movement; select the correct size and repeat the procedure.
9 If the fit is correct secure the joining device or other appropriate head immobilisation device.
10 Ensure that manual in-line cervical stabilisation is maintained until padding and tape is in position.

Application of padding and tape

Equipment (Figure 16.4)

1 Two blankets/pads.
2 Strong narrow tape.

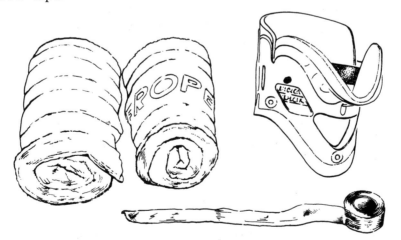

Figure 16.4. Padding, hard collar, and tape

Procedure

1 Ensure that manual in-line cervical stabilisation is maintained by a second person throughout.

2 Place a blanket/pads either side of the head.
3 Apply tape across the forehead and securely attach it to the long spinal board.
4 Apply tape across the chin piece of the hard collar and securely attach it to the long spinal board.

> **Exceptions to the rule**
>
> Both the frightened, uncooperative casualty and the casualty who is hypoxic and combative may paradoxically have increased cervical spine movement if padding and tape are applied. This is because these casualties will fight to escape from any restraint. In such cases a hard collar alone should be applied, and no attempt made to immobilise the head

Sandbags are traditionally used in hospital for head immobilisation. In the pre-hospital setting these should be replaced with rolled up towels, blankets or padding as they produce less forces on the neck during transportation.

Specialised immobilisation equipment

It is often quicker and simpler to use equipment specifically designed for head immobilisation and its use should be encouraged whenever appropriate. It is the pre-hospital carer's responsibility to choose the most appropriate head immobilisation equipment available. If specialised immobilisation equipment is not available or appropriate for the given circumstance, improvisation will be required.

Paediatric spinal boards

There are a number of proprietary boards available for the immobilisation of children with spinal injuries. These generally make securing a child much easier, but remember, trying to tie down a combative child may do more harm than good. If they are combative, try to guide their movements while supporting the head with your hands.

Other equipment

Adult spinal boards are generally too large for children and they tend to slide about and require lots of packing around them. The head hugger should be removed in small children or the neck may be flexed unduly.

For very small children a Kendrick extrication device (KED) makes a very useful spinal board. Strap the child on with their head towards the foot area of the device and simply secure the straps around the patient. Recently, immobilisation of tiny children in large box splints has also been suggested.

Child car seats

If the child is still in a removable car seat then you can leave them in place in the seat (it's an environment they know)—pad around them with towels or blankets and take them safely to hospital.

LOG-ROLLING

In order to minimise the chances of exacerbating unrecognised spinal cord injury, non-essential movements of the spine must be avoided. If manoeuvres which might cause spinal movement are essential (for example during examination of the back during the secondary survey) then log-rolling should be performed. The aim of log-rolling is to maintain the orientation of the spine during turning of the child. The basic requirements are an adequate number of carers and good control.

Procedure

1 Gather together enough personnel to roll the child. In larger children four people will be required; three will be required in smaller children and infants.
2 Place the assistants as shown in Table 16.1.

Table 16.1. Position of assistants during log-rolling

Assistant	Size of child	
	Smaller child and infant	Larger child
1	Head	Head
2	Chest	Chest
3	Legs and pelvis	Pelvis
4		Legs

3 Ensure each helper knows what they are going to do, as shown in Table 16.2.

Table 16.2. Responsibilities of assistants during log-rolling

Assistant position	Task
Head	Hold either side of the head (as for manual in-line cervical stabilisation), and maintain the orientation of the head with the body in all planes during turning. *Control the log-roll by telling other assistants when to roll and when to lay the child back on to the trolley*
Chest	Reach over the child and carefully place both hands over the chest. When told to roll the child, support the weight of the chest and maintain stability. Watch the movement of the head at all times and roll the chest at the same rate.
Pelvis and legs	*This only applies to smaller children and infants. If it is not possible to control the pelvis and legs at the same time, get additional help immediately.* Place one hand either side of the pelvis over the iliac crests. Cradle the child's legs between the forearms. When told to roll the child grip the pelvis and legs and move them together. Watch the movement of the head and chest at all times and roll the pelvis and legs at the same rate
Pelvis	Place one hand either side of the pelvis over the iliac crests. When told to roll the child grip the pelvis and roll it. Watch the movement of the head and chest at all times and roll the pelvis at the same rate
Legs	Support the weight of the legs either by placing both hands under them, or by holding them on each side. When told to roll the child watch the movement of the chest and pelvis and roll the legs at the same rate

APPLICATION OF A LONG SPINE BOARD

There are two common methods of doing this: using a scoop stretcher, or log-rolling. Using a "scoop" is often easiest and safest.

Scoop stretcher

The patient is "scooped" onto the scoop stretcher and the scoop stretcher is used to transfer the patient on to the spine board. Once on the spine board, the scoop stretcher is removed. The scoop stretcher is *not* a substitute for a spine board, as it will tend to flex in the middle. It should therefore be supported during lifting if the child is large.

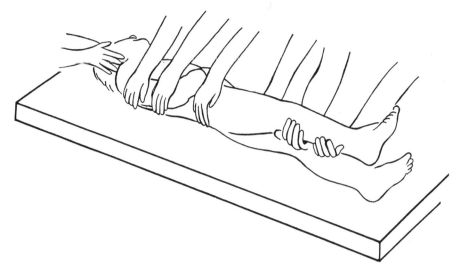

Figure 16.5. Log-rolling a larger child

Log-rolling on to a spine board

Procedure

1 Gently move the head into neutral alignment.
2 Log-roll the casualty (see above).
3 Place the long spine board next to the casualty; the board can be placed flat on the ground, at an angle, or flat against the patient's back, the last minimising the spinal movement, but requiring more rescuers (see Figure 16.6).
4 Log-roll the casualty back on to the board (if the board was against the casualty's back or at an angle to it, the patient and the board are lowered together).
5 Taking care not to cause spinal movement, position the casualty in the centre of the board.
6 Place the casualty's arms by the side.
7 Immobilise the lower body on to the board.
8 Immobilise the legs on the board.
9 Pad under and around the head as necessary, place head blocks (or an alternative such as rolled up blankets) either side of the head, and immobilise by strapping over the forehead and across the cervical collar.

Rapid extrication

> **Rapid extrication is indicated if the scene is unsafe, if the casualty's condition is such that life saving interventions are necessary (and cannot be performed *in situ*), or if the patient is blocking access to a casualty with life threatening injuries**

The technique described is that for a sitting casualty. The exact positioning of rescuers may need to be varied depending on individual circumstances.

Minimum equipment

1 Cervical collar.
2 Long spine board.
3 Straps.

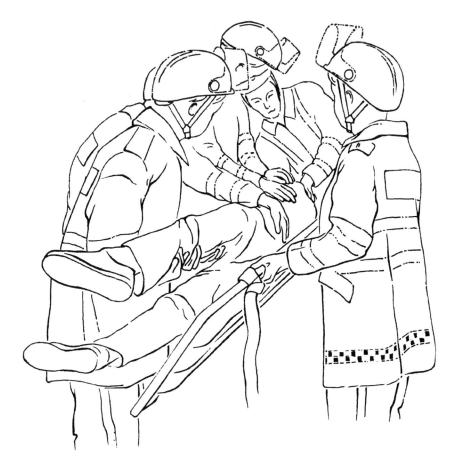

Figure 16.6. Application of a long spine board

Procedure

1 Gather together enough personnel to perform the procedure; a minimum of three people will be necessary.
2 Place the helpers as shown in Table 16.3. This may mean that one or more rescuers are inside a vehicle, building, or other structure.

Table 16.3. Assistant positions during rapid extrication

Assistant	Position
1	Head
2	Left
3	Right

3 The first rescuer brings the head to a neutral position.
4 A second rescuer (the one on the side to which the casualty is to be moved) supports the patient's chest.
5 The casualty is moved to the sitting position.
6 After rapid assessment the cervical collar is applied.
7 A third rescuer (the one on the side away from which the casualty is to be moved) ensures that there are no obstacles preventing movement of the patient's lower body and legs.
8 The casualty is rotated bit by bit (Figure 16.7) until facing away from the desired direction of movement; in-line stabilisation of the cervical spine is maintained throughout (Figure 16.8).

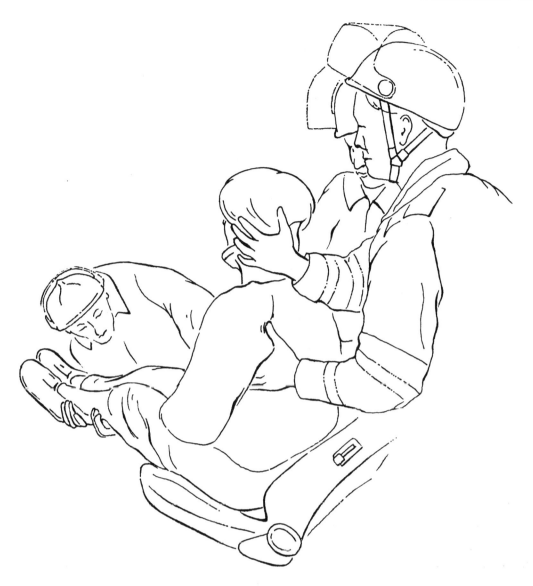

Figure 16.7. Rotating the patient

9   A long spine board is inserted under the upright patient.
10   The patient's upper body is lowered on to the board.
11   While in-line stabilisation is maintained, the patient is slid along the board until centred on it (Figure 16.8).

> **Spinal control will be lost if the complete rotation is carried out in one movement**

HELMET REMOVAL

Cycle or motorcycle helmets must be removed without causing cervical spine movements. This requires a minimum of two people.

1   Obtain a history of the mechanism of injury.
2   Explain the procedure to patient and parent(s).
3   Perform a mini-neurological examination.
4   The first rescuer provides in-line immobilisation by holding the occipital ridge with one hand and placing the thumb and forefinger of the other hand along the mandible.

149

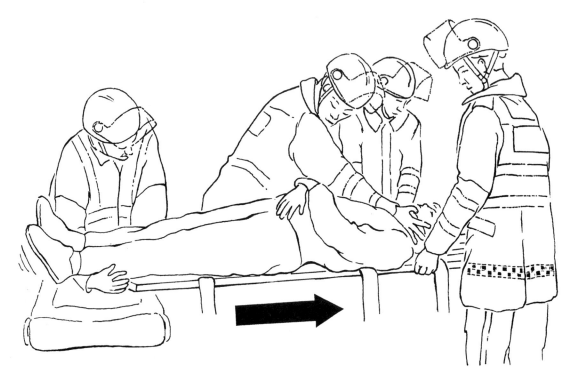

Figure 16.8. On to the spine board

5 The second rescuer opens the face shield (removes specs) and undoes or cuts the chin strap.
6 The second rescuer kneels behind the patient's head and grasps the lower edge of the crash helmet on either side with each hand, spreading it laterally if necessary.
7 The rescuer then rotates the helmet towards himself until the face bar contacts with the patient's nose, then rotates the helmet forward to clear over the patient's occiput.
8 Once the rear of the helmet contacts it may require further lifts of the face bar to clear the nose then the forehead.
9 Remove the helmet over the front of the head.
10 The patient should then be placed in a cervical collar, sandbags and taped to the spine board.*
11 Carry out a brief neurological examination again.

* A restless, agitated child should not be sandbagged and taped because of inducing further cervical spine damage.

FEMORAL NERVE BLOCK

The femoral nerve supplies the femur with sensation and is useful in cases of femoral fracture. Usually a long acting local anaesthetic such as bupivacaine is most useful to allow for splinting and moving the patient, but if a rapid effect is required lignocaine may be used (see Table 16.4). The technique may be useful even when opiates are contraindicated.

Equipment

- Antiseptic swabs.
- Lignocaine 1%.
- 10 ml and 2 ml syringes.
- 25 G and 21 G needles.
- Bupivacaine.

Table 16.4. Drugs in femoral nerve block

Drug	Dose
Bupivacaine 0.5% vol (long acting)	0.3 ml/kg (0.5% vol solution)
Lignocaine 1% (rapid onset)	0.3 ml/kg (1% solution)
CHECK STRENGTH OF DRUG BEFORE GIVING	

Procedure

1 Move the fractured limb gently so that the femur lies in abduction and the ipsilateral groin is exposed.

2 Swab the groin clean with antiseptic solution.

3 Identify the femoral artery and keep one finger on it. The femoral nerve lies immediately lateral to the artery.

4 Using the 2 ml syringe, fill with lignocaine and 25 G needle, infiltrate the skin just lateral to the artery. Aspirate the syringe frequently to ensure that the needle is not in a vessel.

5 Inject the bupivacaine or lignocaine around the nerve using the 21 G needle, taking care not to puncture the artery or vein.

6 Wait until anaesthesia occurs (bupivacaine may take up to 20 minutes to have its full effect).

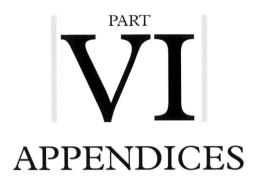

PART

VI

APPENDICES

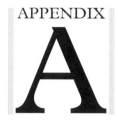

APPENDIX A

Fluid administration

INTRODUCTION

It is uncommon to need to administer intravenous fluids to children in the pre-hospital environment. This chapter aims to cover two of the commonest reasons—shock and hypoglycaemia.

The commonest cause of electromechanical dissociation is reduction in circulating blood volume (hypovolaemia). Knowing how to treat this may be life saving. Distributive shock causes a "relative" hypovolaemia which also requires fluid resuscitation (ie fluid in addition to the normal daily requirements) to maintain the circulation.

Hypoglycaemia may occur in diabetes, as in adults, but children are also very prone to hypoglycaemia from other causes, which are discussed below.

HYPOVOLAEMIC SHOCK

Hypovolaemia is the most common type of shock seen in children. It is due to an inadequate amount of fluid being in the circulation because of:

- Inadequate intake.
- Sudden excessive loss (blood loss, burns, vomiting, diarrhoea).

DISTRIBUTIVE SHOCK

In distributive shock the body has an increased requirement of fluid to maintain the blood volume rather than having lost or failed to replace fluid. There are two main reasons:

- Fluid leaking out of the circulation into the tissues because of "sick" capillaries (septic and anaphylactic shock) or, more rarely, low albumin levels in the blood (protein losing pathologies).
- Vasodilatation, in which relative hypovolaemia may occur. When the blood vessels dilate, the amount of blood within them will suddenly become inadequate to maintain the pressure they were previously maintaining. This occurs in anaphylaxis, sepsis, spinal cord injury, and overdoses of some drugs.

DIAGNOSIS OF SHOCK

A correct diagnosis is necessary to decide treatment.

History

A brief history as to the cause of the patient's problem must be sought. This is needed to confirm the type of shock the patient has, in order to provide the correct treatment.

Physical examination

Evaluation, as always should be by ABC. The physical signs of circulatory failure, as outlined in Table A.1, should be carefully noted, with the exception of blood pressure which may be measured at a convenient later time. Note particularly that the blood pressure falls very late in children. This is why it is not a good guide to initial assessment: if the child is hypotensive, the other, easier to measure signs will be abnormal anyway and are easier to repeat to assess progress.

Table A.1. Assessment of shock

Sign	Percentage blood loss		
	<25	25–40	>40
Heart rate	Tachycardia +	Tachycardia + +	Tachycardia/bradycardia
Systolic BP	Normal	Normal/falling	Falling
Pulse volume	Normal/reduced	Reduced +	Reduced + +
Capillary refill time	Normal/increased	Increased	Increased + +
Skin	Cool/pale	Cold/mottled	Cold/pale
Respiratory rate	Tachypnoea +	Tachypnoea + +	Sighing respiration
Mental state	Mild agitation	Lethargic/uncooperative	Reacts only to pain, or unresponsive

Interpretation of findings

The vital signs of children vary at different ages. These are given in Table A.2. Children have healthy cardiovascular systems which compensate well in adversity, so physical signs must be carefully looked for. The severity of the abnormalities will give a guide to the severity of the shock. **Remember hypotension is a pre-terminal sign**.

Table A.2. Vital signs at different ages

Age (years)	Respiratory rate (breaths/min)	Systolic BP	Pulse (/min)
<1	30–40	70–90	110–160
2–5	25–30	80–100	95–140
5–12	20–25	90–110	80–120
>12	15–20	100–120	60–100

TREATMENT OF SHOCK

At every point of the assessment of ABC give appropriate resuscitation.

Administration of oxygen

This is essential for all types of shock.

156

Drugs

If the child has **anaphylaxis**, adrenaline is the mainstay of treatment, although intravenous fluid may also be needed.

Intravenous fluid

If there is any suspicion that the child may have **cardiogenic shock** (pump failure), usually because he or she has a known cardiac problem. They should be given oxygen but **not intravenous fluids**, because this could make the child worse. They should be rapidly transported in a position of comfort, to hospital.

Intravenous fluid may be given in hypovolaemic or distributive shock when there is a clear sign as to what has caused the shock (visible blood loss, meningococcal purpura) and when the following factors are taken into consideration:

1 Type and cause of shock.
2 Severity of circulatory failure.
3 Ease of vascular access.
4 Journey time to hospital.
5 Personnel and equipment available.

> Remember not to delay transportation while gaining vascular access unless the benefits of the procedure outweigh the detriment of delay

Choice of fluid

Crystalloid or colloid may be used. There are arguments for and against both, which are beyond the scope of this book. Often patients ultimately need a mixture of not only crystalloid and colloid but also blood. If crystalloid is used, a bigger volume will be necessary to re-expand the circulation than if colloid is used. Some crystalloid solutions will provide a sugar source (Table A.3) and so may be the most appropriate if the child is also hypoglycaemic.

Table A.3. Types of crystalloid

Fluid	Comments
"Normal" saline, 0.9% saline	Isotonic with plasma
Various % saline made up with dextrose to make them isotonic. (The more dextrose the less saline)	Can be useful in babies to provide a sugar source to prevent hypoglycaemia
5% dextrose	Isotonic with plasma
Hartmann's solution (also called Ringer's lactate)	Isotonic. Also contains K+ and lactate Does not contain sugar

In the United Kingdom it is more common to use colloid in the first instance, if available, because it stays in the circulation longer. Table A.4 summarises the properties of colloid solutions. If colloid is not available, use crystalloid—preferably one with a significant amount of sodium in it, such as 0.9% saline or Hartmann's solution. Sodium concentrations are given on the side of all bottles or bags. The sodium level in the blood may drop if low sodium solutions are used. In addition, sodium promotes water retention in the body so normal saline (0.9%) is advantageous in the shocked patient.

What route should be used?

Peripheral venous access is preferred and veins may best be in the antecubital fossa or on the medial side of the ankle (see Chapter 15).

Table A.4. Types of colloid

Fluid	Constituents
4.5% human albumin solution	Albumin, buffers
Haemaccel	Gelatine
Gelofusin	Gelatine
Pentastarch	Hydroxyethyl starch

Intraosseous infusion is an excellent technique to use in extremis in children where vascular access cannot be achieved in 90 seconds or two attempts at intravenous access have failed.

Central venous cannulation in the pre-hospital setting is not recommended because it is (a) difficult and (b) takes a long time, during which the child could usually be moved. Intraosseous infusion is much easier, much safer, and much quicker.

How much fluid should be given?

This will depend upon the weight of the child estimated from a standard chart or tape, or using the formula below.

$$\text{Weight in kg} = 2 \, (\text{age in years} + 4)$$

A child's blood volume is 80–100 ml/kg, smaller children having relatively larger volumes. It is usual to start by giving a fluid bolus of 20 ml/kg of fluid. This represents 25% of the child's normal circulating volume and should produce a clinically detectable response. If reassessment of the clinical signs shows that the child is still shocked, then a further 20 ml/kg can be given.

It is crucial that the fluid administered is accurately measured. Most bags/bottles of fluid come as 500 ml minimum. Any child weighing less than 25 kg (an average 8-year-old) should have fluid administered either through an automated intravenous fluid pump or by syringing it in using a syringe and three-way tap in the giving set. Gravity controlled, burette containing giving sets do not generally run well in the back of moving vehicles. They often lead to unnecessarily slow fluid administration and clotted cannulae. If possible, they should be avoided. Fluid should be given as rapidly as possible and ideally should be syringed in.

A good way of documenting syringefuls of fluid is to use a "five bar gate" system on the skin of a convenient part of the child (leg, back of hand etc). An indelible mark or "bar" represents one syringeful (either 20 ml, 50 ml etc). This means the record cannot be lost and the administrator of the fluid cannot lose count—but it is crucial that the receiving unit know how to interpret it, so excellent handover is necessary.

HYPOGLYCAEMIA

This is a common problem in children and must be checked for by a stick test in any child with a disturbed conscious level.

Diabetic hypoglycaemia

This is due to a relative excess of administered insulin to glucose in a diabetic patient. If possible the patient should be treated with oral glucose such as Hypostop, following it up with more substantial carbohydrate when recovered. Intravenous glucose should be given if the oral route is not possible. The weight of the patient should be estimated (see above) and the child given the equivalent of 5 ml/kg of 10% dextrose titrating the dose to the response. **The dextrose concentration must not exceed 20–25%** because high concentrations of dextrose given rapidly can cause brain damage and have even caused death. Because the cause of the hypoglycaemia is excess insulin, not deficient glucose stores, it is reasonable to give IM glucagon to mobilise glycogen from the liver if vascular access is not appropriate. It does, however, cause vomiting and an unpleasant hangover.

Other causes of hypoglycaemia

In all other causes of hypoglycaemia, the blood sugar is low because the child has burnt up all the store in the liver, so glucagon may be ineffective. Oral or intravenous glucose is likely to be required, although glucagon may be tried if no vascular access has been obtained.

SUMMARY

- In managing the shocked child an assessment must be made of the type and severity of shock so that specific therapies are instituted.
- Transportation should not be delayed to gain vascular access unless the situation is life threatening.
- The need for fluid administration will depend on the cause of the shock, the severity, the journey time, the predicted time for vascular access, and the personnel and equipment available.
- Peripheral venous access is preferable but intraosseous access is excellent in emergencies.
- In hypovolaemic shock it does not matter greatly which type of fluid is used, but if crystalloid is used it should contain as close to 0.9% saline as possible.
- A clear record of exact fluid administered should be kept.
- When treating hypoglycaemia, remember glucagon may not work in non-diabetic children.
- Glucose concentrations exceeding 25% should *not* be given to children.
- In all cases where a child has received intravenous/intraosseous fluids, the hospital should be warned of the child's arrival and a very clear handover regarding fluid volume and type administered should be given.

APPENDIX

B

Child protection

INTRODUCTION

All those working with children have an overwhelming impulse to deny that human beings will harm their young. Health care workers will come into contact with:

1 Children who have been abused by adults or by other children.
2 Children who have abused other children.
3 Adults who were abused as children.

In any group of staff up to 10% of people may have been abused themselves. If these survivors have had support following the abuse they will be able to recognise and help abused children. If they have residual problems arising out of their own abuse, they may become disturbed and need help themselves if approached by children or adults whose experiences reflect their own.

Background

The standard of care of children has varied over the centuries. Up to the nineteenth century children were used in industry in a manner which today we would classify as abuse. In Victorian times beating children as a means of discipline was accepted by most social groups. Today corporal punishment is forbidden in schools, but the laws of the United Kingdom allow parents to administer physical punishment to children within prescribed limits.

A good working definition is that **a child is considered to be abused if he or she is treated by an adult or by another child in a way that is unacceptable in a given culture at a given time**.

The extremes of physical abuse were described in 1962 by Kempe, an American paediatrician, as the "battered baby syndrome"—multiple bruises, intracranial haemorrhages, fractures, and internal injuries in children under the age of one year. In Liverpool, between 1978 and 1987, there were five deaths of children under the age of 5 years due to similar injuries.

CLASSIFICATION OF CHILD ABUSE

Since 1962 we have gradually recognised many more forms of abuse. Present classifications are as follows:

Neglect

Neglect means the persistent or severe neglect of a child, or the failure to protect a child from exposure to any kind of danger, including cold or starvation, or extreme failure to carry out important aspects of care, resulting in the significant impairment of the child's health or development, including non-organic failure to thrive. There are at least 20 areas of care in which children may be neglected.

Physical injury

This is actual or likely physical injury to a child, or failure to prevent physical injury (or suffering) to a child, including deliberate poisoning, suffocation and Munchausen's syndrome by proxy.

Sexual abuse

This is the involvement of dependent, developmentally immature children, and adolescents, in sexual activities they do not truly comprehend, to which they are unable to give informed consent or which violate the social taboos of family roles. There are many types of sexual abuse:

- Touching, fondling or licking of genitals or breasts.
- Masturbation of child by adult or adult by child; or of an adult in the presence of the child.
- Body contact with the adult genitals, including rubbing or simulated intercourse by the adult against or between thighs, buttocks or elsewhere.
- Heterosexual or homosexual intercourse with actual or attempted vaginal, anal or oral penetration.
- Exhibitionism (the display of genitals).
- Involvement in pornography, including photography and erotic talk.
- Involvement in prostitution, male or female.
- Other varieties of sexual exploitation.

Most of these abusive acts will leave no physical signs on the victim.

Emotional abuse

This is described as an actual or probable severe adverse effect on the emotional and behavioural development of a child caused by persistent or severe emotional ill treatment or rejection. All abuse involves some emotional ill treatment. This category should be used where it is the main or sole form of abuse.

Grave concern

This is described in children whose situations do not currently fit the above categories, but where social and medical assessments indicate that they are at significant risk of abuse. These could include situations where another child in the household has been harmed or the household contains a known abuser.

Organised abuse

This characteristically involves multiple perpetrators, involves multiple victims, and is a form of organised crime. There are three sub-sections. The first is paedophile and/or pornographic rings. The second is cult-based ritualistic abuse in which the abuse has spiritual or social objectives. The third is pseudoritualistic abuse in which the degradation of children is the end rather than the means.

PRESENTATIONS OF PHYSICAL ABUSE

- Head injuries—fractures, intracranial injury.
- Fractures of long bones
    - single fracture with multiple bruises;
    - multiple fractures in different stages of healing, possibly with no bruises or soft tissue injury;
    - metaphyseal or epiphyseal injuries, often multiple.
- Fractured ribs.
- Spinal injuries.
- Internal damage.
- Burns and scalds.
- Cold injury—hypothermia, frostbite.
- Poisoning—drugs or household substances.
- Suffocation.
- Cuts and bruises—imprints of hands, sticks, whips, belts, bites etc may be present.
- Blindness.

PRESENTATIONS OF SEXUAL ABUSE

- Disclosure by child.
- Suspicion by third party because of behaviour of child, especially changes in behaviour. These include: insecurity; fear of men; sleep disorders; mood changes, tantrums, aggression at home; anxiety, despair, withdrawal, secretiveness; poor peer relationships; lying, stealing, arson; school failure; eating disorders, anorexia, compulsive overeating; running away, truancy; suicide attempts, self-poisoning, self-mutilation, abuse of drugs, solvents, alcohol; unexplained acquisition of money; sexualised behaviour, drawings with a sexual content; knowledge of adult sexual behaviour shown in speech, play or drawing; apparently sexual approaches; promiscuity.
- Symptoms such as a sore bottom, vaginal discharge, bleeding per rectum, inflamed penis which the caregiver believes is due to sexual abuse.
- Symptoms as above and/or signs eg unexplained perineal tear and/or bruising, torn hymen, perineal warts, but doctor is the first person to suspect abuse.
- Sexually transmitted disease.
- Faecal soiling or relapse of enuresis.
- Child (usually adolescent girl) presents frequently with a variety of problems, including recurrent abdominal pain, overdose of drugs, reluctance to go home.
- Pregnancy but girl refuses to name the putative father or even indicate the category, eg boyfriend, casual acquaintance.

CLASSIC POINTERS TO PHYSICAL ABUSE

Classic pointers to the diagnosis of inflicted injury are:

- There is delay in seeking medical help or medical help is not sought at all.
- The story of the "accident" is vague, is lacking in detail, and may vary with each telling and from person to person. Innocent accidents tend to have vivid accounts that ring true.
- The account of the accident is not compatible with the injury observed.
- The parents' affect is abnormal. Normal parents are full of anxiety for the child who has been injured.
- The parents' behaviour gives cause for concern. They may become hostile, rebut accusations that have not been made, or refuse to agree to the child going to hospital.

- The child's appearance and his or her interaction with the parents are abnormal. The child may look sad, withdrawn or frightened. There may be visible evidence of a failure to thrive. Full-blown frozen watchfulness is a late stage and results from repetitive physical and emotional abuse over a period of time.
- The child may disclose abuse. Always listen carefully and record accurately the words of the child.

MANAGEMENT OF DISCLOSED OR SUSPECTED ABUSE

Pre-hospital workers have an unrivalled opportunity to assess the scene. They may be able to see that the injury is not compatible with the history just by looking at the place in which it is said to have occurred. They also have an opportunity to assess the child's home surroundings and environment in a way that hospital personnel cannot. Such information may subsequently be invaluable.

Roles

The roles of the pre-hospital health care professional in child protection are:

- Assess **A**irway (including cervical spine control), **B**reathing, **C**irculation and **D**isability.
- Resuscitate.
- Transport the child to a place of safety, usually a hospital, as soon as is practical.
- Observe the home conditions.
- Observe the child and the inter-relationships within the household.
- Make detailed, legible, signed records of all observations.
- Pass on these observations to the person taking over the care of the child.

If the parents are refusing medical care, the situation should be discussed with a paediatrician, preferably one experienced in child protection. Many areas of the UK now have specialised units with staff designated for this work. Doctors in these units are on call for advice to all health care professionals and colleagues in other disciplines. Accident and Emergency Department staff are also available to discuss concerns. If the situation is violent, the police should be contacted.

The child who has disclosed abuse or who is the subject of suspected abuse will be overwhelmed by the number of professional people who will be involved in the assessment of the situation. If the disclosure or suspicion arises in a nursery or school, then teachers and health visitors/school nurses will make preliminary enquiries and referrals. In all intra-familial abuse social workers will speak to the child and the family. They will be responsible for the safety of the child, for ongoing care of the family, and for any subsequent civil proceedings. All child abuse is criminal activity so police officers will interview the alleged victim, the alleged offender, and any other witnesses to the incidents. In most areas of the UK good liaison exists between social workers and police officers so joint interviews are done to minimise the number of times the child will have to relate the details of the incident(s). Whenever possible, these interviews are recorded on videotape to be used as evidence. Under the Criminal Justice Act 1991 videotapes can be used as evidence in chief for children under the age of 14 years, provided that the child is available for cross-examination.

The medical assessment should be done by a paediatrician with forensic training or jointly by police surgeon and a paediatrician. If the child has severe psychological disturbance or psychiatric symptoms then a psychologist and/or psychiatrist should also see the child and the family.

Each person should be very careful not to abuse the child further by overlapping with the roles of the other professions.

MEDICOLEGAL ASPECTS

Health care professionals must be familiar with the medicolegal aspects of their work. The most important are the following:

- Emergency Protection Orders, Police Protection Orders.
- Consent to examination.
- Writing of statements and reports for criminal and civil proceedings.
- Presentation of evidence.

Emergency Protection Order (EPO)

The Emergency Protection Order (Children Act 1989, sections 44 and 45) replaced the Place of Safety Order. It may be made for a maximum of 8 days with a possible further extension of up to 7 days. An application for discharge of that order may be made. The court may only make the order if it is satisfied that there is reasonable cause to believe that the child is likely to suffer significant harm if either he is not removed to another place or if his removal from a safe place (such as a hospital) is not prevented. Another clause is that in the case of an application made by a Social Services Department or the NSPCC, the applicant "has reasonable cause to suspect that a child is suffering or is likely to suffer significant harm" and enquiries which are being made with respect to the child "are frustrated by access to the child being unreasonably refused" and the applicant believes that access is required as a matter of urgency.

Police Protection Order

A constable has powers (Children Act 1989, section 46) to take a child "into police protection" for up to 72 hours. This power can be used to move a child from home to a hospital or to another place of safety.

Consent to examination

Consent for all examinations which are for evidential purposes must be obtained from a person with parental responsibility. In the Children Act 1989 (section 3) parental responsibility is defined as "all the rights, duties, powers, responsibilities and authority which by law a parent has in relation to the child and his property". Those with parental responsibility are specified in the Children Act 1989 (section 2). This can be summarised as in Box B.1.

Box B.1 PARENTAL RESPONSIBILITY

- Parents married at time of birth. Both have parental responsibility which continues after separation or divorce
- An unmarried mother has parental responsibility
- An unmarried father can apply to obtain parental responsibility; he can be appointed a guardian or if he can prove paternity then he can have the same legal position as if married
- Person in whose favour a Residence Order has been made—this is for the duration of the Order
- Appointed guardian
- Local Authority while a Care Order is in force
- Person who applies for an Emergency Protection Order

When more than one person has parental responsibility, each can act alone and without the other in meeting that responsibility. Parents do not lose parental responsibility if a Care Order or an Emergency Protection Order is in force. Parents lose parental responsibility with an Adoption Order. Parental responsibility can be delegated to a person acting on their behalf, eg while they are on holiday.

To cover emergency situations, those caring for a child who do not have parental responsibility may do what is reasonable in all the circumstances for the purpose of safeguarding or promoting the child's welfare.

Consent from the child or young person is needed if that person is of sufficient understanding to make an informed decision. Lawyers suggest that in a normal child this would be at age 10 years. The Gillick ruling (1986) allows an individual under the age of 16 years to submit to examination and treatment without the parents being informed, provided that is the wish of the child or young person.

Court reports

Anyone who has had contact with a family in which abuse is disclosed or suspected may be asked to give evidence in civil or criminal proceedings. When preparing a written report on a child for the court all health care professionals should keep in mind that the written report may be used in subsequent court appearances. Therefore, the report should be confined to the facts. Whenever possible, objective and measurable evidence of the home circumstances, and the child's health and development should be presented. Where subjective views must be given they should reflect balanced professional judgement. If the report is comprehensive and comprehensible, then the health care professional may not be called to give verbal evidence in person. Always keep a copy of the report and a photocopy of the original notes if they have to be filed in a general filing system. All court personnel will ask for the original notes to be produced, but if these have gone missing then a photocopy may be acceptable. For the health care professional this is essential for good evidence.

Statements

The purpose of a statement is to provide the court with an informative and relevant account of the contact which that person had with the child and the family. The statement will give details of the persons involved, the observations and findings. Information given by another person should not be included unless this has been requested. In many areas the Crown Prosecution Service wish statements to record all information, although hearsay may be excluded before presentation to the court.

A statement is a professional document. It should be well written in good basic English. Technical terms should be avoided or if quoted should be followed immediately by appropriate lay terms. Most statements will be for the prosecution and a printed statement form will be provided. The standard sequence of writing a statement is as shown in Box B.2.

Box B.2   SEQUENCE FOR WRITING STATEMENTS

 1 Full name with surname in capitals
 2 Qualifications
 3 Occupation
 4 Name of person requesting the report
 5 Date, time, and place of contact with the child
 6 Name of child
 7 Name of persons present
 8 Details of the relevant history
 9 Details of examination
10 Treatment given
11 Opinion on findings
12 The time at which contact with the child ended
13 Date the report is made

Each page of the statement must be signed at the bottom and the final page must be signed on the line below the completion of the writing. Any alterations must be initialled. Always keep a copy of the statement.

Presentation of evidence

Dress in a professional manner. Arrive early in court. Take along all notes relevant to the case. Read these on the day before the court proceedings. With permission from the magistrate or judge, you may refer to contemporaneous notes. However, revision helps to put the whole picture of the incident into the forefront of your mind so that you can find the appropriate notes more quickly.

When giving evidence stay calm, even if the barrister becomes aggressive or even abusive. Do not be persuaded to answer questions which are outside your knowledge or experience. When answering questions, try to speak directly to the bench, not to the barrister.

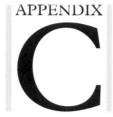

C

Childhood accidents and their prevention

INTRODUCTION

Child accident and injury prevention is important because:

- On average, two children die in accidents every day.
- Accidents are the commonest cause of death among children age 1–14 years.
- They cause half of all deaths of children aged between 10 and 14 years.
- Accidents result in about 10 000 children being permanently disabled annually.
- Accidents cause one child in five to attend an Accident and Emergency Department every year.
- Accidents lead to one-fifth of all hospital paediatric admissions.

To put it another way, accidental injury to children leads to about 468 deaths, 120 000 hospital admissions and about 2 million Accident and Emergency Department attendances in England and Wales every year.

This is the bad news about children's accidents. The good news is that they may often be prevented. Accidents are not unpredictable acts of God; they are closely linked to the child, their circumstances and their development. There are measures available that can prevent accidents completely or diminish their impact, measures which are applicable to a variety of fields.

RISK FACTORS

Who is most at risk? There are definite predisposing factors which enable high risk groups to be identified.

Sex

Boys are more frequently injured than girls. The difference emerges at age 1–2 years. How much of this difference is innate and how much cultural is a subject for speculation. Girls may mature more rapidly in terms of perception and coordination.

Age

Children's accidents are intimately related to development. Take falls as an example. A newborn baby can only fall if dropped, or if a parent falls holding the baby. An older baby can wriggle and roll off a changing table or a bed. A crawling baby can climb upstairs and fall back. A small child can climb and fall out of a window. An older child can climb a tree, or fall in a playground. Knowledge of development helps anticipate dangers.

Exposure to different circumstances also varies with age. Children under 5 years experience accidents at home. School age children experience accidents at school, sport and play, and are especially at risk of accidental deaths as pedestrians.

Social class

As with so many other health problems, accidents are linked to inequalities in environments. Children in social class V (as derived from head of household's occupation), are twice as likely to die from an accident as children in social class I, and for some accident types, such as burns, the chances are six times higher.

This does not mean that working class parents care less about their children than middle class parents, or they do not know about accident risks. It may mean that there are many other pressures—overcrowding, lack of money, poor housing—and there is less power—owning one's own home, being able to afford safety equipment—to make changes for safety.

Psychological factors

Accidents are more common in families where there is stress from mental illness, marital discord, moving home, and a variety of similar factors.

Ethnic origin

On the whole, social class is more important than ethnic origin in determining accident risk.

ACCIDENT PREVENTION

How can injuries be prevented? There are a number of basic principles.

Accidents can be prevented **completely**. This is termed primary prevention. An example is a fireguard preventing access to an open fire. The harm caused by an accident can be **minimised**. This is secondary prevention. For example, a seatbelt can reduce injury even if a car crash occurs. Finally, rapid attention to an injury can **reduce mortality and morbidity**. This is tertiary prevention. Examples are cold water on burns and scalds or pressing on a laceration.

There are three main approaches to accident prevention. These are the following:

- **Education**
  Increasing knowledge about a problem and the solutions, to change attitudes and eventually behaviour.
- **Engineering**
  Safe design of products and the environment, including the architecture of the home.
- **Enforcement**
  The role of legislation, regulations, and standards in accident prevention.

Countermeasures can be active, that is a conscious decision to use them has to be taken every time, such as putting pans on the back hobs of the cooker. Or, they can be passive, that is, built in to the product: for example, junior formulations of paracetamol are sold in small bottles that do not contain a lethal dose.

There are a variety of ways in which doctors and other health care personnel can participate in reducing children's injuries.

- **Be informed**

  This can be at a personal level. Many professionals could learn more about child safety from a Mothercare catalogue than they did as part of undergraduate or postgraduate education. Suggestions for reading are included.

- **Set a good example**

  Wear your seatbelt. Drive carefully past schools. Consider your own home and family with safety in mind.

- **Take opportunities**

  Can you offer safety advice to a family after an accident has happened? Do you know possible preventative strategies for that accident type? Have you developed the communication skills to listen to parents, and advise them? Can you photograph that injured child in that setting, and use it to support a family in improving their household, or a neighbourhood in a media campaign?

- **Collaborate with others**

  Be prepared to participate in working groups and campaigns. You have special expertise and influence to offer.

Children's accidents and injuries are the major public health problem to children in Britain today. All health care workers can learn more about them, and have something to offer in reducing their toll.

SUGGESTED READING

JG Avery and RH Jackson (1993) *Children and their accidents*. Hodder & Stoughton. Available from bookshops. ISBN 0–340–37001–7.
Professor IB Pless (1993) *The scientific basis of childhood injury prevention—A review of the medical literature*. Child Accident Prevention Trust. Available by post from CAPT, 4th Floor, 18–20 Farringdon Lane, London EC1R 3AU. (Price £6.00 inc. post and packing.)

D

Dealing with death

As already stressed, the outcome for attempted resuscitation for cardiorespiratory arrest in childhood is poor. This is particularly so in out-of-hospital arrest and in the case of "cot death" where the infant is usually not discovered until resuscitation is impossible.

All those involved in pre-hospital care are likely to have to cope with the sudden death of a child. This can lead to great stress and those involved should be supported in this aspect of their work by being taught about it beforehand and by staff counselling sessions afterwards.

Parental presence during cardiopulmonary resuscitation is becoming increasingly common. The important thing is that the parents should have the choice whether to be there or not. In an ideal situation a health care professional should be available exclusively for the support of the parents but in most out-of-hospital situations this will not be practical because the same personnel will be doing both the resuscitation and supporting the parents. This adds to the great stress which is engendered by the death of a child.

If the child has been the victim of an accident and the injuries have resulted in disfigurement or deformity there is a natural tendency to protect the parents from seeing their child. Usually parents can handle severe injuries. The uppermost thought in their minds is to be with their child, to hold his or her hand, and to give last hugs. Many parents complain that they were overprotected by health care workers and regret that they were denied what they considered to be precious last moments with their child. Often the confirmation of death is not done in an out-of-hospital situation because a doctor is not available, but in extreme circumstances, eg when rigor mortis has occurred, no resuscitation attempts will be made. If the decision that the child is dead or appears to be dead has been made then this should be told to the parents as soon as possible. The news should be broken sympathetically and without euphemisms. If it is appropriate and the person breaking the news is comfortable doing it, sympathy can be shown by holding the parent's hand or by putting an arm around the parent. In many situations, although the pre-hospital carers suspect that death is inevitable, they will attempt resuscitation during the journey to hospital. Always refer to the child by name and under no circumstances refer to him or her as "it".

Most deaths in infancy and childhood are due to natural causes or accidents but occasionally infanticide or homicide does occur. Careful notes should be made of any unusual circumstances in the home or at the scene from which the child was moved to hospital. This information may be very valuable to any investigation by the police on behalf of the coroner, who is always informed of sudden unexpected deaths.

Always transport the child to hospital even if you have confirmed that the child is dead. The reasons for this are that a full history, investigations, and proper counselling of the parents are essential. In a few areas of the country there may be exceptions to this guidance and local protocols should be known by those involved in pre-hospital care. Inform the hospital of the expected time of arrival and whether resuscitation is being attempted. Generally the child should be taken into the resuscitation room and not certified in the back of the ambulance.

During the journey to hospital, transport the child as you would a patient who is alive. The parents may wish to hold their baby. No child should ever be transported in a black bag. The parents should be allowed to look at the child in the ambulance. Ensure that both parents or one parent and a relative or friend are available to support each other. Give advice on practical issues, eg care of other children, locking the house and taking keys to hospital. Be prepared to handle any reaction—silence, shouting, numbness, and crying are all normal reactions to a suspicion or knowledge that a child is dead or dying. At all stages be very careful what you say to the parents. Chance remarks linger in the memory.

Be aware of any personal difficulties which you have in handling death and bereavement and get support or counselling for this, preferably before another similar situation arises.

Dealing with death

The child

- Attempt cardiopulmonary resuscitation unless death is certain
- Transport the child on a stretcher or in the arms of a parent
- Always transport the child to hospital unless local protocols advise otherwise
- Always refer to the child by name and the appropriate gender

The parents

- Explain that the child appears to have died—or has died if qualified to say so
- Allow parents to be with their child if they so wish on the journey to hospital
- Allow two adults to accompany the child if practical
- Advise on care of other children, locking the house and taking keys etc
- Always be gentle, unhurried, calm, and careful in the words that you use
- Remember that many reactions in the acute stage of bereavement are normal

Yourself

- Inform the hospital of the expected time of arrival and whether resuscitation is being attempted
- Be aware of any personal difficulties you may have in handling the death of a child and obtain support beforehand and by staff counselling sessions afterwards

---

APPENDIX

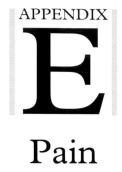

Pain

INTRODUCTION

In general, children, particularly very young ones, are under-treated for pain. This is all the more so in the pre-hospital environment where a number of extra compounding problems exist in addition to those encountered in hospital.

These may include:

- lack of easy access to the patient (eg entrapment);
- difficulty in estimating the size of the child and thus the analgesic dose;
- personnel encountering children infrequently, who thus may be relatively inexperienced in paediatrics and paediatric procedures (eg cannulation);
- fear and logistical difficulties of carrying narcotic analgesics outside hospital;
- delay in obtaining specialist medical help (flying squad, anaesthetist) rapidly on scene.

In addition, the more general reasons for under-treatment of pain will also apply, such as:

- fear of side effects—respiratory depression, airway obstruction with vomiting etc;
- failure to accept that children, especially infants, feel pain like adults;
- the child's fear of needles;
- fear of masking symptoms, eg head injured child, abdominal symptoms.

Inadequate analgesia can be detrimental in the critically ill child. Bronchoconstriction and increased pulmonary vascular resistance caused by pain can lead to hypoxia, worsening shock. Management may also be more difficult—for example, in entrapment and extrication situations.

RECOGNITION AND ASSESSMENT OF PAIN

There are four main ways in which we recognise that a child is in pain:

- A description from the child or parent.
- Behavioural changes such as crying, guarding of the injured part, facial grimacing.
- Physiological changes such as pallor, tachycardia, and tachypnoea which are observed by the clinician.
- An expectation of pain because of the pathophysiology involved, eg fracture, burn or other significant trauma.

172

It must also be remembered that young children localise pain poorly and they have a great potential for masking pain. Remember, therefore, in the injured child, to always look carefully for other trauma—and never forget the cervical spine. The purpose of pain assessment is to establish, as far as possible, the level of pain relief required.

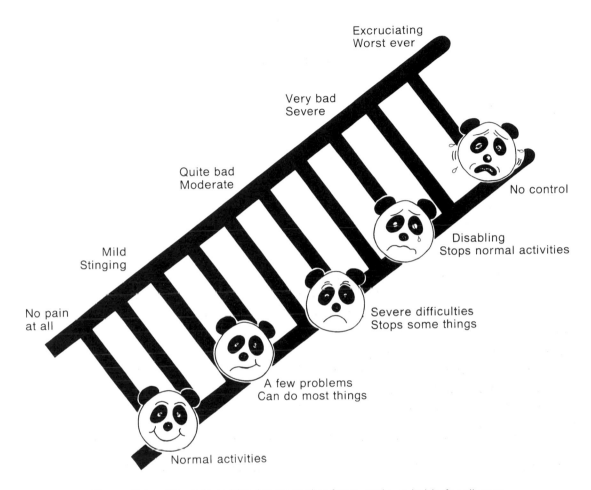

Figure E.1. The pain ladder, incorporating faces scale, suitable for all ages

Detailed pain scale assessment in hospital using validated scales of the type used in hospital (Figure E.1) may not, however, always be practical in the pre-hospital environment and "best guess" may be more practical.

Non-pharmacological methods of pain relief

Environment

Fear worsens pain: the environment may range from the security of the child's home to the roadside or playground. Although the environment may be difficult to control, every effort should be made to protect paediatric patients from other horrific sights and hysteria. Parents and carers should be told that they can best help the child by remaining calm and reassuring and not be hysterical. Care should also be taken that other onlookers are not making the child more frightened either by what they say—or even by staring—and their presence should be discouraged unless they are contributing positively. Once inside the ambulance, attempts should be made to make it as child friendly as possible—evidence of invasive instruments (eg needles) should be minimised. Injuries should be covered where possible.

173

Physical treatments

1 *Distraction* The presence of parents is important. In one study almost all children between the ages of 9 and 12 reported that "the thing that helped most" was to have a parent present during a painful procedure. If it is explained to the parent that they can help most by being reassuring and remaining with the child, it will have the added benefit of making the parents feel they are "doing something" at a time when most parents feel unbelievably helpless. Allow and encourage touching, such as hand holding, particularly if it is not possible for the child to see the parent easily, such as when the cervical spine is immobilised. (Where possible, in this common situation, take care to explain to the parent that the child can only see straight upwards, so that if logistics allow, the parent can bend right over the child to allow them to see their face.) Parents (or other carers) should participate in other distracting strategies such as looking at a book or toy with the child.

2 *Tasks* Simple tasks such as holding the Entonox mask may be not only distracting but provide a degree of control for the child. Parents can again participate in simple tasks such as this, holding an oxygen mask near the face etc.

3 *Reassurance* As stated above, fear worsens pain. Children may fear many things following, for example, an accident, ranging from (sometimes quite reasonably) death, fear of hospitals, needles and what is to come, to parent separation or even loss of a favourite bit of clothing. This is, partly, but not entirely age-dependent. Reassure spoken fears and try to anticipate non-verbalised fears. As with an adult, always provide reassurance if an ambulance siren is to be used—older children will fear the worst and any child in whom it is necessary is unlikely to be well enough to find it "fun".

Never lie to children, particularly if you are going to hurt them. They will never trust you, or indeed any other medical personnel again. The one exception to this is if a child asks if they are going to die in acute emergency—it is important to remain positive and reassuring.

4 *Immobilisation* As with adults, immobilisation of fractures, dislocations etc can provide excellent pain relief. Some dislocations may be reduced if suitably trained personnel are available. Remember to tell the child if you are going to hurt them and why, before doing so.

Pharmacological methods of pain relief

These can be divided into local anaesthetics, non-opiate and opiate analgesics and anaesthetic agents used as analgesics.

Local anaesthetic agents

Topical anaesthetics EMLA (eutectic mixture of local anaesthetics containing lignocaine and prilocaine) and Ametop (amethocaine gel) are topical anaesthetics which are applied under an occlusive dressing prior to venepuncture. The dressing has to be left in place for at least 20 minutes, limiting their use in the emergency pre-hospital setting. However, serious consideration should be given to pre-hospital personnel applying such a dressing over a suitable vein if elective venepuncture is thought to be likely on arrival in hospital.

Infiltrated local anaesthetics These are again of limited use to provide regional nerve blocks before hospital because of the specialist skill required to administer them. They are, however, extremely effective at providing regional analgesia if such personnel are available, and administration does not unduly delay transport, as may sometimes be the case with femoral nerve blocks.

Non-opiate analgesics

1 *Paracetamol:* This is a mild analgesic with antipyretic properties and is very safe in the recommended dose and very dangerous in overdose. It can be given orally or rectally but has a long onset to action (about 30 minutes).

2 *Ibuprofen and diclofenac:* These non-steroidal anti-inflammatory drugs are slightly more potent than paracetamol in analgesic effect (particularly diclofenac) and also have a long onset action. Both can be given orally and diclofenac, rectally. They should be avoided in asthmatics. Aspirin is contraindicated in children aged less than 12 years.

Opiate analgesics:

1 *Morphine* is the standard for analgesia against which all other opiates are measured. It is a potent analgesic which produces some euphoria. It also causes a dose related respiratory depression. Morphine seems to produce less nausea and vomiting in children than in adults.

2 *Diamorphine* is twice as potent as morphine and produces similar effects. It is less commonly used in children.

3 *Nalbuphine* is commonly used in the pre-hospital setting, because, unlike morphine and diamorphine, its use is not controlled under the Misuse of Drugs Act, 1971. It is, however, less potent, causes less euphoria, and still causes respiratory depression. As it is a partial morphine antagonist, it may also potentially interfere with further analgesia given in hospital.

Parenteral opiates should always be given intravenously or via the intraosseous route as absorption from the intramuscular route is very unreliable. All three drugs can produce respiratory depression and therefore should only be used by personnel competent in paediatric airway and breathing assessment and management. They are all also reversible with naloxone, which always should be available when opiates are used. Concurrent administration of anti-emetics should not be routine in children as they tend to cause more side effects than in adults. Furthermore, young children seem to have less problems with vomiting with opiates than adults.

Anaesthetic agents used as analgesics

1 *Entonox:* This is a mixture of 50% nitrous oxide with 50% oxygen and is usually supplied using a demand valve, ie the valve only operates when the patient inhales and applies a negative pressure. This means the patient has to be awake and cooperative. It takes 2–3 minutes to take effect and in addition to being analgesic is quite dissociative. Entonox can be used in any child old enough to cooperate with its administration and children aged 5 or younger may manage it if suitably supported. The black rubber masks can be frightening and can either be replaced with a mouthpiece attachment or the transparent silicone masks. ("Flavoured" versions of these are now obtainable.) Entonox must not be used in children with possible intracranial or intrathoracic air leaks since replacement of the air by Entonox may increase the pressure.

2 *Ketamine:* Ketamine is an anaesthetic agent which can be given either intramuscularly or intravenously which produces analgesia/anaesthesia in about 30 seconds intravenously and 3–4 minutes intramuscularly. In normal doses it does not produce respiratory depression or loss of pharyngeal or laryngeal reflexes although increased

salivation may occur. Temporary elevation of blood pressure is common (although hypotension is not unknown). Vivid dreams and hallucinations are common, but are less troublesome in children than adults. Because of its general anaesthetic effect, ketamine is usually only administered by doctors skilled in airway management (often anaesthetists). In complex, prolonged, and severely painful or frightening situations, ketamine may be invaluable, even if it is necessary to bring a doctor skilled in its use to the scene to administer it. It should be avoided in patients with raised intracranial pressure.

Table E.1. Drugs used in pain control

Analgesic	Pain severity	Dose	Duration of effect	Common side effects	Comments
Paracetamol	Mild	Over 3 mth: 15 mg/kg orally or rectally	4–6 h		Avoid in liver impairment
Ibuprofen	Mild/ moderate	5 mg/kg orally	4–6 h	Avoid in asthmatics	Not for patients <10 kg
Diclofenac	Moderate	1 mg/kg orally or rectally	8 h	Avoid in asthmatics	Not for patients <1 year
Morphine	Moderate to severe	Over 1 yr: 0.1–0.2 mg/kg 3 mth to 1 yr: 0.05–0.1 mg/kg	2–4 h	Respiratory depression Hypotension	Monitor respiration ECG Pulse oximetry
Ketamine	Severe/ entrapped	0.25–4 mg/kg IV 6–13 mg/kg IM	Dose dependent up to about 30 min	Salivation Hallucinations	General anaesthetic Use with atropine and consider concurrent benzodiazepine

Choice of analgesic

In addition to the severity of pain, there are a number of logistical issues which have to be considered when choosing an analgesic in the pre-hospital setting. Is it possible to approach the patient safely? Are opiates available on the scene or will they have to be obtained from elsewhere? Can adequate airway management be provided should the airway or breathing become compromised by over-sedation? Is intravenous access possible? Time from the hospital is a further consideration. Is it "worth" getting a specialist doctor to come and give excellent analgesia or, bearing in mind that transportation should not be delayed in paediatric emergencies, will the child be in the Accident and Emergency Department by the time the doctor arrives?

The following questions need to be addressed:

1 *How severe is the pain?* This can be assessed as outlined above
2 *What analgesia is available?* This will vary. Remember that the simple, non-pharmacological methods of pain relief are available to all. The route of drug administration, side effects, availability of antidotes, and experience of the personnel administering it will all need to be considered.
3 *How long will it take to get to hospital?* Is the child trapped—if so how long will it take to free him or her? The time from the hospital may affect the choice of analgesia. Remember that some analgesics (particularly EMLA and mild/moderate analgesics given orally) may take a long time to be effective, whereas Entonox is effective in a couple of minutes.

4   *Must the analgesia be given before leaving the scene (delaying the on scene time)?* Non-pharmacological, psychological methods of pain relief should be an integral part of patient management from the time medical help arrives. Physical methods of pain relief such as simple splinting of fractures, slings etc are also part of standard patient care. The indications for pharmacological interventions before moving the patient are much more limited. Only life saving interventions should delay transportation, but occasionally it may be too painful to move the patient without analgesia. Obtaining vascular access will prolong the on-scene time and the benefits must outweigh the disadvantages of delay. If possible, Entonox should be used (if not contraindicated) and definitive intravenous pain relief given, if required, once access is established en route to hospital.

5   *Does the time it takes to remove the child to hospital and the severity of the pain merit bringing a suitably skilled doctor to the scene?* This will depend on the severity of the pain and the length of time it will take for the doctor to reach the scene. Remember that transportation should not be delayed unless the benefits outweigh the risks of delay. The usual situation would be that of a trapped child, where the on-scene time is unavoidably prolonged, allowing the medical staff time to reach the scene before the child is released.

6   *Are there any methods of pre-emptive pain control which can be started prior to hospital?* If possible the child should be given some idea as to what might happen in hospital: "They will want to take some pictures of your leg—it won't hurt." This may reduce the fear of the unknown. In addition, consideration should be given as to whether a local anaesthetic cream should be applied over a vein, if it is thought venepuncture may be likely.

SUMMARY

- Pain control is at least as important in children as adults.
- Non-pharmacological methods are available to all and should be an integral part of patient care.
- Pharmacological methods will depend on the individual situation.
- Pre-emptive pain control should always be considered, prior to hospital arrival.

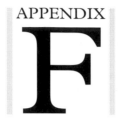

F

Resuscitation of the newborn

The resuscitation of newborn babies is different from the resuscitation of all other age groups and a knowledge of the relevant physiology and pathophysiology is essential. However, the majority of newborn babies will establish normal respiration and circulation spontaneously.

NORMAL PHYSIOLOGY

After delivery of a healthy term baby, the first breath usually occurs within 60 seconds of clamping or obstructing the umbilical cord. Clamping of the cord leads to the onset of asphyxia which is the major stimulant to start respiration. Physical stimuli such as cold air or physical discomfort help provoke respiratory efforts. The first breaths are especially important as the lungs are initially full of fluid.

Labour causes the cells within the lung which secrete lung fluid to cease secretion and begin reabsorption of that fluid. During vaginal delivery up to 35 ml of fluid is expelled from the baby's lungs by uterine contraction. In a healthy baby the first spontaneous breaths generate a negative pressure of between $-40\,cmH_2O$ and $-100\,cmH_2O$ (-3.9 and $-13\,kPa$) which inflate the lungs for the first time. This pressure is 10–15 times greater than that needed for later breathing when the lungs are aerated but is necessary to overcome the viscosity of fluid filling the airways, the surface tension of the fluid-filled lungs and the elastic recoil and resistance of the chest wall, lungs, and airways and the resistance of the airways. These powerful chest movements cause fluid to be displaced from the airways into the lymphatics.

Neonatal circulatory adaptation commences with the detachment of the placenta but lung inflation and alveolar distension releases mediators which affect the pulmonary vasculature as well as increasing oxygenation.

Surfactant (which is 85% lipid) is made by the type II (granular) pneumocytes in the alveolar epithelium. Surfactant reduces alveolar surface tension and prevents alveolar collapse on expiration. Surfactant can be demonstrated from 20 weeks' gestation, but the increase is slow until a surge in production at 30–34 weeks. Surfactant is released at birth due to aeration and distension of the alveoli. The half-life of surfactant is approximately 12 hours. Production is reduced by hypothermia (<35 °C), hypoxia and acidosis (pH <7.25).

PATHOPHYSIOLOGY

Acute asphyxia deprives the body of oxygen. Initially breathing becomes deeper and more rapid, but if unsuccessful the baby loses consciousness quite quickly and increasing hypoxia causes cessation of breathing within 2–3 minutes (primary apnoea) (Table F.1). Babies have a number of automatic reflex responses to such a situation: energy is conserved by shutting down the circulation to all but vital organs such as the heart, lungs, and brain. Bradycardia ensues but blood pressure is maintained by peripheral vasoconstriction and increased stroke volume. After a latent period of primary apnoea, which may vary in duration, spinal gasps ensue. These deep spontaneous gasps are easily distinguishable from normal respirations as they occur 6–12 times per minute and involve all accessory muscles in a maximal inspiratory effort. After a while even this activity ceases (terminal apnoea) (Table F.1) and the most primitive medullary reflexes are extinguished. The time taken for such activity to cease is longer in the newborn than in later life, taking up to 20 minutes.

Table F.1. Assessment of the newborn

	Healthy	Primary apnoea	Terminal apnoea
Colour	Pink	Blue	Blue/white
Respiration	Regular	Irregular or inadequate	Absent
Heart rate	>100/min	>100/min	<100/min

The circulation is almost always maintained until all respiratory activity ceases. This resilience is a feature of all newborn mammals, largely due to the reserves of glycogen in the heart. Resuscitation is therefore relatively easy if undertaken before all respiratory activity has stopped. Once the lungs are inflated, oxygen will be carried to the heart and then to the brain. Recovery will then be rapid. **Most** infants who have not progressed to terminal apnoea will resuscitate themselves if their airway is patent.

Once gasping ceases, however, the circulation starts to fail and these infants are likely to need extensive resuscitation.

Meconium

Hypoxia in the term infant (>37 weeks) leads to gut vessel vasoconstriction, increased peristalsis, and a relaxation of the sphincters. This leads to meconium passage in utero. In addition, fetal hypoxia as described above leads to gasping and aspiration of amniotic fluid with meconium.

Once the baby is delivered, meconium causes problems related to complete or partial airway obstruction. With the asphyxial insult this combines to produce a multi-organ problem which is fortunately relatively uncommon in the UK.

Slight coloration of liquor with meconium is not significant.

PRACTICAL ASPECTS OF NEONATAL RESUSCITATION

The basic approach to resuscitation is **Airway**, **Breathing**, and **Circulation** but there are a number of additions to the formula:

- Get help
- Note the time
- Dry, wrap, and keep baby warm
- Assess baby
- Then:
  Airway
  Breathing (lung inflation and ventilation)
  Circulation
  Drugs

179

Call for help

Always ask for help if you expect or encounter any difficulty.

Note the time

If possible/available.

Temperature control

Dry the baby off immediately and then wrap in a dry towel. A cold baby has an increased oxygen consumption and cold babies more easily become hypoglycaemic and acidotic. They also have an increased mortality. If this is not addressed at the beginning of resuscitation it is often forgotten. Most of the heat loss is by latent heat evaporation—hence the need to dry the baby. There is also a large surface area to weight ratio thus heat can be lost very quickly. Ideally pre-hospital delivery should take place in a warm room or a warmed ambulance. However, drying effectively and wrapping the baby in a warm towel is the most important factor in avoiding hypothermia. A naked wet baby can still become hypothermic despite a warm environment. One of the biggest problems in pre-hospital delivery is hypothermia.

Assessment of the newborn

Acute assessment is made by examining:

- **Colour**   (pink, blue, white).
- **Heart rate**   (palpation, auscultation).
- **Respiration** (rate and quality).

This will categorise the baby into one of the three following groups:

1   *Pink, regular respirations, heart rate >100/min*
    These are healthy babies and they should be kept warm and given to their mothers.

2   *Blue, irregular or inadequate respirations, heart rate >100/min*
    If gentle stimulation does not induce effective breathing, the airway should be opened and cleared. If the baby responds, then no further resuscitation is needed. If not, progress to lung inflation.

3   *Blue or white, apnoeic, heart rate <100/min*
    Heart rate and colour will give some indication of whether the baby is in primary or terminal apnoea (Table F.1) but this is not always obvious. The management is the same initially with control of the airway followed by lung inflation. A reassessment of the heart rate then directs further resuscitation. A response at any stage should prompt reassessment.

The Apgar scoring system (Table F.2) was proposed as a tool for evaluating a baby's condition at birth. Although the score, calculated at 1 and 5 minutes, may be useful retrospectively it is often subjective and it is not used to guide resuscitation.

Table F.2. Apgar scoring

Score	Heart rate	Respirations	Muscle tone	Reflex irritability (catheter in nares)	Colour
0	Absent	Absent	Limp	No response	Blue or pale
1	Slow (<100/min)	Slow, irregular	Some flexion	Grimace	Pink body with blue extremities
2	>100/min	Good, crying	Active motion	Cough or sneeze	Completely pink

White colour, apnoea and low or absent heart rate are indicators of profound perinatal asphyxia. However, management of such babies is unchanged but may be prolonged. Depending upon the assessment, resuscitation follows:

Airway
Breathing
Circulation
Drugs

Airway

The baby should be positioned with the head in the neutral position. Over-extension may collapse the newborn's airway at the back of the pharynx more than under-extension. Beware the large occiput—a folded towel placed under the neck and shoulders may help to maintain the airway in a neutral position and a jaw thrust may bring the tongue forward. Gentle suction of nares and oropharynx with a soft suction catheter may stimulate respiration. Blind deep pharyngeal suction should be avoided as it may cause vagally induced bradycardia and laryngospasm.

Meconium

Although a major worry, this is fortunately very uncommon. If meconium or any airway obstruction is suspected and the baby has not yet breathed, the upper airway should be visualised directly using a laryngoscope and any particulate matter suctioned. If meconium is found the baby should be intubated, if possible, and the trachea suctioned using suction applied to the endotracheal tube as it is withdrawn slowly. Suction must not exceed -70 mmHg (-9.8 kPa) and is applied briefly and intermittently. This may be repeated until resuscitation can be continued. If intubation is not possible, continue with resuscitation.

Breathing (inflation breaths and ventilation)

The first 5–6 breaths should be inflation breaths. These should be 2 second sustained breaths. Use a transparent, circular, soft mask big enough to cover the nose and mouth of the baby. A 500 ml self-inflating bag with a reservoir bag and a blow-off valve set at 30–40 cmH$_2$O should be employed.

The chest may not move during the first 1–3 breaths as fluid is displaced. Once the chest is inflated, reassess the heart rate.

Once the chest is inflated, ventilation is continued at a rate of 30–40 per minute.

Circulation

The easiest place to feel the pulse is at the base of the umbilical cord.

Once the lungs are inflated, cardiac compressions must be started if the rate is still below 80/min. The most efficient way of doing this in the neonate is to encircle the chest with both hands, so that the fingers lie behind the baby and the thumbs are apposed on the sternum just below the inter-nipple line. Briskly compress the chest trying to halve the distance between your fingers and thumbs. **Give three compressions to each inflation.**

The purpose of cardiac compression is to move oxygen or drugs to the coronary arteries in order to initiate cardiac recovery. There is no point in cardiac compression before the lungs have been aerated.

Once the heart rate is above 80/min, and rising or >100/min, cardiac compression can be discontinued.

Drugs

If after adequate aeration, oxygenation, ventilation, and cardiac compression the heart rate has not responded, drug therapy should be considered. Vascular access is best via an umbilical venous line, but although easy, this is not always available in the pre-hospital setting. In this case adrenaline can be given down the endotracheal tube at a dose of 20 mcg/kg. If the umbilicus cannot be catheterised, the intraosseous route *can* be used in newborns.

1 *Adrenaline*
    In the presence of profound unresponsive bradycardia or circulatory standstill, 10 mcg/kg (0.1 ml/kg 1:10 000 adrenaline) may be given intravenously or endotracheally. Further doses of 10–30 mcg/kg (0.1–0.3 ml 1:10 000 adrenaline) may be tried at 3–5 minute intervals if there is no response. The endotracheal route is accepted but unproven in neonatal resuscitation.

2 *Bicarbonate*
    In the presence of circulatory stasis there will be profound acidosis as it occurs in terminal apnoea (Table F.1). Acidosis depresses cardiac function and adrenaline does not bind to receptors in a highly acidotic cardiac milieu. Bicarbonate 1 mmol/kg (2 ml/kg of 4.2% solution) is used to change that milieu and enhance the effects of oxygen and adrenaline. Bicarbonate remains controversial and should only be used in the absence of discernible cardiac output or profound and unresponsive bradycardia.

3 *Glucose*
    Hypoglycaemia is a potential problem for all stressed or asphyxiated babies. It is easily and safely treated by using 5 ml/kg of 10% dextrose intravenously. BM stix are not reliable in neonates when reading less than 5 mmol/l.

4 *Colloid*
    Very occasionally hypovolaemia may be present because of known or suspected loss (antepartum haemorrhage, placenta or vasa praevia, unclamped cord) or be secondary to loss of vascular tone following asphyxia. Colloid 20 ml/kg may be required.

5 *Naloxone*
    This is not a drug of resuscitation. Occasionally a baby who has been effectively resuscitated and is pink with a heart rate over 100 per minute, may not breathe because of the effects of maternal opiates. If respiratory depressants' effects are suspected the baby should be given naloxone 200 mcg intramuscularly in a full-term baby. Smaller doses of 10 mcg/kg will also reverse the sedation but the effect will only last a short time (20 minutes IV or a few hours IM). Atropine and calcium have no place in neonatal resuscitation.

RESPONSE TO RESUSCITATION

Often the first indication of success will be an increase in heart rate. Recovery of respiratory drive may be delayed. Babies in terminal apnoea will tend to gasp first as they recover before starting normal respirations. Those who were in primary apnoea are likely to start with normal breaths, which may commence at any stage of resuscitation.

TRACHEAL INTUBATION

Most babies can be adequately resuscitated using a mask system. Swedish data suggest that if this is applied adequately, only 1 in 500 babies actually need intubation. However, endotracheal intubation remains the gold standard in airway management. It is especially useful in prolonged resuscitation, pre-term babies, and meconium aspiration. It should be considered if mask ventilation has failed, although the most common reason for failure with mask inflation is poor positioning of the head with consequent failure to open the airway.

The technique of intubation is the same for infants and is described in Chapter 14. A normal full-term newborn usually needs a 3.5 mm endotracheal tube, but 2.5 and 3.0 mm tubes should also be available.

PRE-TERM BABIES

The more pre-term a baby, the less likely it is to establish adequate respirations. Pre-term babies (<32 weeks) are likely to be deficient in surfactant. Work of respiration will be increased although musculature will be less developed. One must anticipate that babies born before 32 weeks may need help to establish prompt aeration and ventilation. Pre-term babies with surfactant deficiency may need relatively higher inflation pressures than term babies. Pre-term babies are more likely to get cold (higher surface area to mass ratio), and more likely to be hypoglycaemic (fewer glycogen stores).

ACTIONS IN THE EVENT OF POOR INITIAL RESPONSE TO RESUSCITATION

1 Check airway and breathing.
2 Check for a technical fault:
    (a) Is oxygen connected?
    (b) Is mask ventilation effective? Auscultate both axillae and observe movement.
    (c) Is endotracheal tube in the trachea? Auscultate both axillae and observe movement.
    (d) Is endotracheal tube in the right bronchus? Auscultate both axillae and observe movement.
    (e) Is endotracheal tube blocked?
    If there is any doubt about the position or patency of the endotracheal tube it must be replaced.
3 Does the baby have a pneumothorax? This occurs spontaneously in up to 1% of newborns but those needing action at birth are exceptionally rare. Auscultate the chest for asymmetry of breath sounds. If a tension pneumothorax is thought to be present clinically, a 21 G butterfly needle should be inserted through the second intercostal space in the mid-clavicular line. Alternatively, a 22 G cannula may be used connected to a three-way tap. Remember that you may well cause a pneumothorax during this procedure.
4 Does the baby remain cyanosed but breathing with a good heart rate? There may be a congenital heart malformation preventing normal oxygenation at the lungs or persistent pulmonary hypertension of the newborn. These babies need urgent transfer.
5 If the baby is pink with a good heart rate, it may be suffering the effects of maternal opiates. In this situation naloxone 200 mcg IM may be given. This should outlast the opiate effect, although continued observation is necessary.
6 Is there severe anaemia or hypovolaemia? In the face of large blood loss, 20 ml/kg colloid should be given.

DISCONTINUATION OF RESUSCITATION

The outcome of a baby with no cardiac output after 15 minutes of resuscitation is likely to be very poor. The decision to discontinue resuscitation should be taken by senior medical personnel. This will often be after arrival in hospital.

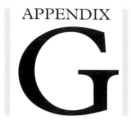

Paediatric triage

> **Definition**
>
> Triage is the process of sorting multiple casualties into priorities for treatment

INTRODUCTION

A recent study looking back over 30 years has revealed that major incidents occur in the United Kingdom on average three or four times per year, and up to 11 times per year. The evidence confirms that the majority of major incidents do involve a proportion of children, and a number of incidents predominantly or exclusively involve children.

There are two identifiable approaches to managing an incident that involves injured children. Some would argue that *all* children should be given the highest treatment priority (Priority 1, IMMEDIATE). After all, every child is dependent to some degree. While this approach can be understood, the danger is that the limited hospital paediatric resources will be diluted, and key personnel will be unavailable to treat the genuine child in need. Additionally, it is difficult to argue rationally why a child should be treated before a more seriously injured adult.

The alternative approach is to prioritise children according to their clinical need, in parallel with adults who have been injured.

METHODS OF TRIAGE

Triage can be anatomical, physiological, or a mixture of the two. Anatomical methods rely on assigning a priority according to the injuries that are evident on physical examination. This has a number of inherent problems:

- The patient must be undressed, which is both time consuming and impractical outside hospital.
- Triage will be inconsistent between observers, depending on their clinical experience.
- Some life threatening conditions will be missed by clinical examination alone—for example, haemoperitoneum is only detected in 35% of cases by examination of the abdomen.

Physiological methods assess the consequences of injury. They have been shown to be simple, safe, rapid and reproducible between observers. These are the preferred methods of triage pre-hospital. The principal disadvantages of these methods are:

- The majority are based on adult physiological parameters.
- In the early period following injury there will be physiological compensation, leading to under-triage.

Mixed methods allow clinical experience to influence the physiological triage priority. Again, this will introduce inconsistency when there are observers with a range of clinical experience.

WHEN TO TRIAGE

Triage is appropriate whenever the number of casualties exceeds the immediate medical resources. It is a dynamic process, and must be repeated at every link of the evacuation chain. Children can be expected to get better or worse at any time.

Importantly, in a multiple casualty situation the rescuer must not attempt to predict how the patient's condition may change. This will inevitably lead to over-triage, and a disproportionate number of Priority 1 and Priority 2 casualties.

SYSTEMS OF TRIAGE

A widely used physiological triage system in the United Kingdom (both civilian and military) and Australia is the **triage sieve**. This uses a simple algorithm to assess mobility, followed by a rapid assessment of ABC. Specifically, there is a need to count the respiratory rate and the pulse (Figure G.1).

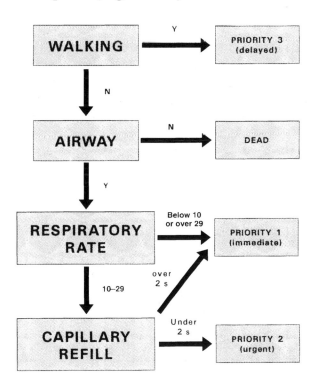

Figure G.1. Triage sieve

However, the **triage sieve** uses adult physiological parameters. For this reason the system has been modified to produce the **paediatric triage tape** (Figure G.2).

The length of a child is proportional to its weight and age. This principle is already exploited in the Broselow tape which relates a child's length to the correct dose of a resuscitation drug (such as adrenaline), or piece of equipment (such as an endotracheal tube). In the same way, the length of a child can be related to the normal physiological parameters for that age. This is the foundation of the paediatric triage tape.

The tape is a series of triage sieve algorithms with respiratory and pulse rates corrected for the length (and age and weight) of the child. The mobility assessment is necessarily

185

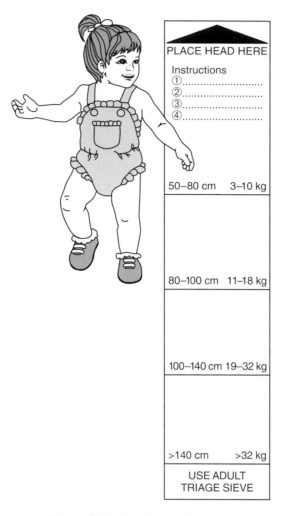

PLACE HEAD HERE

Instructions
① ....
② ....
③ ....
④ ....

50–80 cm   3–10 kg

80–100 cm   11–18 kg

100–140 cm 19–32 kg

>140 cm   >32 kg

USE ADULT
TRIAGE SIEVE

Figure G.2. Paediatric triage tape

different, with an infant being assessed as "mobile" if he or she is moving all limbs spontaneously. Additionally, the capillary refill time (CRT) is only to screen for a normal circulation. If the CRT is delayed, a pulse must still be taken. Children cool quickly, and CRT may be falsely delayed in the cold.

It is recommended that the forehead be used to take the CRT in children. The limited experimental evidence on CRT shows that the only normal distribution of values is when it is performed on the forehead or the sternum (but the sternum requires exposing pre-hospital). The nail bed and the heel produce inconsistent results.

When the tape cannot be used in a trapped child then the child is automatically a Priority 1. Once extrication is complete, the triage priority is reassessed using the tape alongside the child.

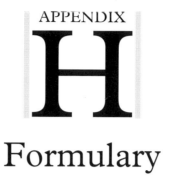

APPENDIX

Formulary

The formulary is intended as a reference to be used in conjunction with this book. To this end, the drugs mentioned elsewhere are set out alphabetically below, along with their routes of administration, dosage, and some notes on their use.

GENERAL GUIDANCE ON THE USE OF THE FORMULARY

The total daily dose of drugs is given. To calculate the actual dose given at each administration, divide the total daily dose by the number of times per day that the drug is to be given.

When dosage is calculated per kilogram and a maximum dose is not stated, then the dose given should not exceed that for a 40 kg child.

The exact dose calculated per kilogram may be difficult to administer because of the make-up of formulations available. If this is the case the dose may be rounded up or down to a more manageable figure.

Doses in the formulary are sometimes written as mcg or ng. When prescribing such doses these terms should be written in full (micrograms or nanograms respectively) in order to avoid confusion.

More detailed information about individual drugs is available from manufacturers, from hospital drug information centres, and from the pharmacy departments of children's hospitals.

ABBREVIATIONS

The following abbreviations are used:

IM	intramuscular
IV	intravenous – all IV drugs can be given IO
SC	subcutaneous
via ETT	via the endotracheal tube
IO	intraosseous

> **The final responsibility for delivery of the correct dose remains that of the health professional prescribing and administering the drug**

Drug	Route	Total daily dose (TDD) 1 month to 12 years	<1 month	Times daily (divide TDD by this figure)	Notes
Adrenaline Injection 1:10 000 Minijet	IV	0.1 ml/kg of 1:10 000 (10 mcg/kg) to a maximum dose of 10 ml of 1:10 000	0.1 ml/kg of 1:10 000 (10 mcg/kg)	First dose (Resuscitation)	α and β sympathomimetic *Ventricular fibrillation, asystole and electromechanical dissociation.* IV doses may be given by intraosseous route flushed with 0.9% saline
		1 ml/kg of 1:10 000 (100 mcg/kg)	0.1–0.3 ml/kg of 1:10 000 (10–30 mcg/kg)	Subsequent doses (Resuscitation)	
Injection 1:1000 ampoules	via ETT	0.1 ml/kg of 1:1000 (100 mcg/kg)	0.1 ml/kg of 1:1000 (100 mcg/kg)	First and subsequent doses (Resuscitation)	Given via endotracheal tube
	IM	0.01 ml/kg of 1:1000 (10 mcg/kg)	0.01 ml/kg of 1:1000 (10 mcg/kg)	Single dose	*Acute anaphylaxis* Dose may be doubled and repeated
	IV infusion	0.05–2 mcg/kg/min	0.05–2 mcg/kg/min	Continuous	Anaphylaxis if bolus dose is not effective
Use injection solution in nebuliser	Nebuliser	5 ml of 1:1000	Use only with advice	Single dose	Airway Management Dilute with 0.9% saline if required, for nebulisation. Repeat every 2–4 hours. Monitor ECG
		Inactivated by sodium bicarbonate			
Atropine sulphate Injection 100 mcg/ml Minijet	IV	20 mcg/kg (minimum 100 mcg)	Do not use in neonates	Single dose	Antimuscarinic *Bradycardia* If increased vagal activity administer over 1 minute. IV doses may be given via the intraosseous route; 40 mcg/kg may be given via endotracheal tube
Benzylpenicillin Injection 600 mg vials 600 mg = 1 megaunit = 1 000 000 units	IV infusion	300 mg/kg to a maximum dose of 12 g		6	Antibiotic (penicillin) *Dose for severe infection*
			Up to 7 days 30 mg/kg	2	Infuse over 30 minutes to reduce irritation and CNS toxicity
			Over 7 days 45 mg/kg	3	Do not mix with aminoglycosides, flush line, or separate by 30 minutes
		See also dose in text Chapter 10, Table 10.3			
		Reduce dose in severe renal impairment, risk of convulsions			
Budesonide	Nebuliser	**Over 3 months** 0.5–2 mg	Do not use in neonates	2	*Croup* Can be mixed with salbutamol and ipratropium

continued

Note: Dose given is total daily dose unless otherwise stated.
If a maximum dose is not stated the dose given should not exceed that for a 40 kg child.

Drug	Route	Total daily dose (TDD) 1 month to 12 years	<1 month	Times daily (divide TDD by this figure)	Notes
Bupivacaine (plain) Injection 0.25% (2.5 mg/ml)	Local infiltration	Up to 2 mg/kg (0.8 ml/kg) to a maximum of 150 mg (60 ml of 0.25%)	Up to 2 mg/kg (0.8 ml/kg)	Single dose not more than every 8 hours	Local anaesthetic See also Chapter 16 for dose for femoral nerve block
		Avoid or reduce dose in liver disease			
Cefotaxime Injection 500 mg, 1 g, 2 g vials	IV	100 mg/kg to a maximum dose of 2 g **then** 200 mg/kg to a maximum dose of 12 g		Initial dose **then** Subsequent doses 4	Antibiotic (cephalosporin) Severe infection Given by short infusion Given by short infusion
			Up to 7 days 100 mg/kg **Over 7 days** 150 mg/kg	Infection 2 3	
		Reduce dose in severe renal impairment. Bolus over 3–5 minutes or dilute 4–10 times with infusion fluid and administer over 20–60 minutes. Do not mix with aminoglycosides			
Chlorpheniramine Injection 10 mg/ml	IV	**1 month– 1 year** 250 mcg/kg **1–5 years** 2.5–5 mg **6–12 years** 5–10 mg to a maximum of 20 mg	Do not use in neonates	Single dose Single dose Single dose	Sedative antihistamine Repeat up to four times in 24 hours if necessary. Dilute with 5–10 ml water for injection or 0.9% saline and give over 1 minute. May cause transient drowsiness, giddiness and hypotension especially if administered too rapidly
Dexamethasone Injection dexamethasone phosphate 8 mg in 2 ml (equivalent to 6.7 mg base in 2 ml); 4 mg in 1 ml (equivalent to 3.3 mg base in 1 ml) All doses are quoted as base	IV	800 mcg/kg 600 mcg/kg		4 Single dose	Corticosteroid–glucocorticoid Meningitis to reduce meningeal inflammation and incidence of severe hearing loss. Usually given for 4 days. Bolus over 3–5 minutes. Infusion in 5% dextrose or 0.5% saline *Croup:* inhaled budesonide may also be used
		Reduces effects of rifampicin and antiepileptics; antagonises effects of diuretics and antidiabetics.			

continued

Note: Dose given is total daily dose unless otherwise stated.
If a maximum dose is not stated the dose given should not exceed that for a 40 kg child.

Drug	Route	Total daily dose (TDD) 1 month to 12 years	<1 month	Times daily (divide TDD by this figure)	Notes
Diazepam Injection 5 mg/ml ampoules In lipid emulsion for injection 5 mg/ ml ampoules	IV	250–400 mcg/kg	200 mcg/kg	Single dose	Benzodiazepine Slow IV bolus over 3–5 minutes. Repeat after 10 minutes if necessary
Rectal solution 5 mg/2.5 ml 10 mg/2.5 ml	Rectal	**Up to 1 year** 2.5 mg **1–3 years** 5 mg **4–12 years** 5–10 mg to a maximum dose of 10 mg	2.5 mg	Single dose Single dose Single dose	Repeat dose if necessary after 5 minutes
		Caution: in liver disease, may precipitate coma. Reduce dose in severe renal impairment. Beware respiratory depression in acute use—antagonist flumazenil. Enhanced sedative effects with anaesthetics, opioid analgesics, isoniazid, antihistamines, α-blockers, antihypertensives, baclofen, ulcer healing drugs, omeprazole. Seek advice			
Diclofenac	Oral/rectal	1 mg/kg		single dose	Avoid asthmatics and children <1 year
Flumazenil Injection 100 mcg/ml ampoules	IV	**Up to 1 year** 50 mcg **1–7 years** 100 mcg **7-12 years** 150 mcg to a maximum dose of 200 mcg then	Do not use in neonates	Single dose	Benzodiazepine antagonist Initial dose over 15 seconds
		Up to 1 year 25 mcg **1–7 years** 50 mcg **7–12 years** 75 mcg to a maximum dose of 100 mcg	Do not use in neonates	Single dose	Repeat dose to be given at 1-minute intervals to maximum dose of 1 mg
		Limited experience in children. Doses quoted for children are derived from adult dose and mean surface area. Contraindicated in prolonged benzodiazepine use in epilepsy			

continued

Note: Dose given is total daily dose unless otherwise stated.
If a maximum dose is not stated the dose given should not exceed that for a 40 kg child.

Drug	Route	Total daily dose (TDD) 1 month to 12 years	<1 month	Times daily (divide TDD by this figure)	Notes
Hydrocortisone					
Injection 100 mg (as sodium succinate = Efcortesol)	IV (IM)	4 mg/kg	2.5 mg/kg	Single dose	Corticosteroid Initial dose
(as sodium phosphate = Solucortef)		2–4 mg/kg	2 mg/kg	Single dose	Maintenance dose. Repeat every 6 hours. Slow IV over 1–5 minutes. May be mixed with 5% dextrose or 0.9% saline.
Ipratropium bromide					Antimuscarinic bronchodilator
Nebuliser solution 250 mcg/ml (100 mcg in 0.4 ml) [prescribe in 25 mcg (0.1 ml) multiples]	Nebuliser	**Up to 7 years** 125 mcg **Over 7 years** 250 mcg	Do not use in neonates	3–4	Nebuliser solution may be diluted with 0.9% saline and/or mixed immediately before use with other nebuliser solutions except sodium cromoglycate
Atrovent 20 mcg/activation, Atrovent Forte 40 mcg/activation	Oral inhalation (aerosol)	Up to 160 mcg/day (8 puffs)	Do not use in neonates	3–4	Inhaler may be used with Nebuhaler (with mask for young children)
		Dry mouth, urinary retention, constipation can occur			
Ketamine		See Appendix on Pain Control			
Lignocaine					*Ventricular fibrillation or tachycardia*
Injection 20 mg/ml (2%) Minijet	IV	1 mg/kg to a maximum dose of 50 mg	1 mg/kg	Single dose	If necessary repeat every 5 minutes to maximum 3 mg/kg. IV dose may be given by the intraosseous route; 2 mg/kg may be given via endotracheal tube
Injection 5 mg/ml (0.5%) 10 mg/ml (1%) 20 mg/ml (2%) ampoules	IV	0.5–1 mg/kg to a maximum dose of 100 mg	0.5–1 mg/kg to a maximum dose of 100 mg	Single dose	*Antiarrhythmic* Loading dose. Administer over 1 minute
	IV infusion	10–50 mcg/kg/min	10–50 mcg/kg/min	Continuous	Maintenance dose. Infuse in 5% dextrose or 0.9% saline at a concentration of 2 mg/ml
	Local infiltration	Up to 3 mg/kg	Up to 3 mg/kg	Single dose not more than every 4 hours	*Local anaesthetic* See also Chapter 16 for dose in femoral block
		Avoid or reduce dose in severe liver disease. Several drug interactions including increased myocardial depression with other anti-arrhythmics, β-blockers. Effect antagonised by hypokalaemia, eg with loop and thiazide diuretics. Metabolism inhibited by cimetidine. Seek further advice			

continued

Note: Dose given is total daily dose unless otherwise stated.
If a maximum dose is not stated the dose given should not exceed that for a 40 kg child.

Drug	Route	Total daily dose (TDD) 1 month to 12 years	<1 month	Times daily (divide TDD by this figure)	Notes
Morphine Injection 2.5 mg/ml 10 mg/ml ampoules	IV	**1–3 months** 0.025 mg/kg	0.025 mg/kg	Single dose	Opiate Repeat up to 4 times in 24 hours
		3–12 months 0.05–0.1 mg/kg		Single dose	Repeat up to 4 times in 24 hours
		Over 1 year 0.1–0.2 mg/kg		Single dose	Repeat up to 6 times in 24 hours
Causes constipation and nausea. Avoid in moderate renal impairment and in liver disease (can precipitate coma). **Caution:** enhances sedative effects of anxiolytics and hypnotics; antagonises effects of cisapride and metoclopramide. Morphine levels increased by cimetidine. Can cause respiratory depression. Antagonist is naloxone					
Naloxone Injection 20 mcg/ml 400 mcg/ml	IV	10 mcg/kg	10 mcg/kg	First dose	Opiate antagonist Give higher dose if response to first dose is inadequate
		then <20 kg 100 mcg/kg	**then** 100 mcg/kg	**then** Single dose	Repeat doses as necessary to maintain opioid reversal. May be given IM, SC or by intraosseous route if IV not possible
		>20 kg 2 mg		Single dose	
	IV infusion	8–30 mcg/kg/hour	8–30 mcg/kg/hour	Continuous	Half-life of opioid may be longer than that of naloxone. Consider infusion in 5% dextrose or 0.9% saline at concentration 4 mcg/ml. Adjust rate as required
Paracetamol					Analgesic and antipyretic Repeat if necessary after 4–6 hours
Suspension 120 mg/5 ml, 250 mg/5 ml Tablets 500 mg Dispersible tablets 500 mg Suppositories 60 mg 125 mg 250 mg 500 mg	Oral or rectal	**1–2 months** Do not use **2–3 months** 10–15 mg/kg **Over 3 months** 15 mg/kg to a maximum dose 0.5–1 g	Do not use in neonates	Single dose Single dose	
Avoid large doses in liver disease—dose-related toxicity					
Salbutamol					Selective β-adrenoceptor stimulant. Bronchodilator
Nebules 2.5 mg in 2.5 ml, 5 mg in 2.5 ml	Nebuliser	**Up to 6 months** Do not use **6 months to 5 years** 2.5 mg **Over 5 years** 5 mg	Do not use in neonates	Single dose	Repeat up to 8 times per day. Dilute to 3–4 ml with 0.9% saline. May be mixed with ipratropium, beclomethasone, budesonide, or sodium cromoglycate nebuliser solutions

continued

Note: Dose given is total daily dose unless otherwise stated.
If a maximum dose is not stated the dose given should not exceed that for a 40 kg child.

Drug	Route	Total daily dose (TDD) 1 month to 12 years	<1 month	Times daily (divide TDD by this figure)	Notes
Inhaler and Autohaler 100 mcg per activation	Oral inhalation (aerosol or powder)	**Up to 6 months** Do not use **6 months to 2 years**	Do not use in neonates		Maximum acute treatment doses. Infants and children less than 2 years should use large volume spacer with mask, 2–5 years a large volume spacer is recommended, 5–12 years a
Ventodisk 200 mcg, 400 mcg powder for use in Diskhaler	Oral inhalation (aerosol or powder)	Up to 2400 mcg **3–4 years** Up to 3600 mcg **Over 5 years** Up to 7200 mcg		6 6 6	spacer, dry powder or autohaler
Rotacaps 200 mcg, 400 mcg powder for use with Rotahaler	Oral inhalation (aerosol or powder)	**Up to 7 years** 200–400 mcg **Over 7 years** 200–600 mcg	Do not use in neonates	Single dose Single dose	Emergency initial treatment doses A maximum of 400–600 mcg can be given in 4 hours A maximum of 800–1200 mcg can be given in 4 hours
					100 mcg via a large volume spacer can be administered every few seconds until improvement occurs. Use a mask for very young children
Injection 500 mcg/ml ampoules	IV	4–6 mcg/kg	Use only with advice	Single dose	Status asthmaticus or hyperkalaemia Bolus injection over 5–10 minutes. Repeat if necessary
Injection for infusion 1 mg/ml ampoules	IV infusion	0.1–1 mcg/kg/min	Use only with advice	Continuous	Infusion in 5% dextrose or 0.9% saline at a concentration of 10 mcg/ml. Doses have been doubled

Caution: potentially serious hypokalaemia, especially in severe asthma. Potentiated by theophylline, diuretics, corticosteroids, hypoxia. Efficacy under 18 months of age uncertain

Sodium bicarbonate					Alkylating agent
Injection 8.4%	IV	1 mmol/kg (1 ml/kg of 8.4%)	1 mmol/kg (1 ml/kg of 8.4%)	Single dose	*Acidosis and hyperkalaemia* Dilute to 4.2% with 0.9% saline or water for injection
1 mmol/ml Minijet		1 mmol/kg (1 ml/kg of 8.4%)	1 mmol/kg (1 ml/kg of 8.4%)	Single dose	*Asystole* Dilute to 4.2% in 0.9% saline or water for injections

Administer slowly. Inactivates sympathomimetics such as adrenaline, dopamine

Note: Dose given is total daily dose unless otherwise stated.
If a maximum dose is not stated the dose given should not exceed that for a 40 kg child.

Answers to questions

CHAPTER 2: WHY TREAT CHILDREN DIFFERENTLY?

1 The weight of a child can be calculated by the formula (age in years + 4) × 2. Answer 24 kg.
2 Uncuffed endotracheal tubes are used in pre-pubertal children in order to avoid oedema round the cricoid ring.
3 Parents may provide reassurance and explanation and keep the child calm. Parents may also participate in treatment—for example, a child may tolerate an oxygen mask when it is held by a parent, but not if it is strapped on the face or held by the doctor or paramedic. Parents should always be involved and understand the situation—a reassured parent will go a long way to reassuring the child.

CHAPTER 3: EXAMINING SICK CHILDREN

1 The following may be observed in assessing breathing in a child:
Unusual position
Recession
Use of accessory muscles
Nasal flaring
Grunting
Tachypnoea
Respiratory rate
2 The following abnormal postures may be noted in a sick child:
Stiff posture (hypertonia) (including neck retraction and back arching (opisthotonus))
Floppiness (hypotonia)
Decerebrate posture
Decorticate posture
3 Toddlers are wary of strangers and new experiences. They can also be particularly wilful and stubborn.

CHAPTER 4: SCENE MANAGEMENT

1 Control of the scene is the first priority at an incident, followed by assessment—safety, quick history, reading the wreckage etc. Secondly, communicate with other services, control and the hospital. Finally, casualties can be triaged and treated in the correct order.
2 Injured children can cause emotions to cloud rational judgement leading to poor decision making.
3 If there is more than one casualty, decisions will have to be made in order to prioritise treatment. Triage will therefore be necessary.

CHAPTER 5: TRANSPORT OF CHILDREN

1 The five elements of pre-hospital patient care are:
Primary assessment
Resuscitation
Secondary assessment
Emergency treatment
Definitive care
2 Definitive care can only be provided at the receiving hospital.

CHAPTER 6: BASIC LIFE SUPPORT

1 The letters **SAFE** stand for **S**hout for help, **A**pproach with care, **F**ree from danger, **E**valuate ABC.
2 The recommended position for a head tilt in an infant is the neutral position and in a small child, the sniffing position.
3 To clear an obstructed airway in an infant back blows and chest thrusts are recommended, and in a child, back blows, chest thrusts, and abdominal thrusts.

CHAPTER 7: ADVANCED SUPPORT OF THE AIRWAY AND VENTILATION

1 (a) The size of the internal diameter of an endotracheal tube can be estimated by the formula (age in years/4) + 4
  (b) The length (cm) of an endotracheal tube at the mouth can be estimated by the formula (age in years/2) + 12
2 A size 2 laryngeal mask airway is appropriate for a 4-year-old child (a 4-year-old weighs [age + 4] × 2 = 16 kg).
3 A self-inflating bag should always have a reservoir bag attached during resuscitation because the inspired oxygen concentration is increased from a maximum of about 50% to at least 90%.

CHAPTER 8: THE MANAGEMENT OF CARDIAC ARREST

1 The commonest cardiac arrest rhythm in children is asystole.
2 The initial dose of adrenaline is 10 mcg/kg (0.1 ml/kg 1 : 10 000) and the subsequent doses are 100 mcg/kg (0.1 ml/kg 1 : 1000). Ten times the dose is used endotracheally. When a rhythm changes and a new protocol is used, it is necessary to return to the initial dose (10 mcg/kg) of adrenaline.
3 The first two shocks are given at a dose of 2 J/kg. Subsequent shocks are given at 4 J/kg. If the protocol is re-entered, shocks commence at 2 J/kg again.

CHAPTER 9: RECOGNITION OF THE SERIOUSLY ILL CHILD

1 The normal respiratory rate for a 4-year-old child is 25–30 breaths per minute.
2 The best place to test capillary refill is on the forehead or chest.
3 The injury is most likely to be on the same side as the dilated pupil.

CHAPTER 10: THE STRUCTURED APPROACH TO THE SERIOUSLY ILL CHILD

1 The primary survey is concerned with the assessment of vital signs, while the secondary survey is concerned with assessing immediately treatable illnesses once vital signs are stable.
2 The distance from the hospital will influence the treatment (including procedures) given. It may also influence the outcome, particularly in cardiac arrest.
3 The following are symptoms of circulatory failure:
Breathlessness
Poor feeding
Sweatiness
Drowsiness
Floppiness
Palpitations
Fluid loss

CHAPTER 11: TREATING SERIOUSLY ILL CHILDREN

1 The child with viral croup should be kept calm and reassured.
2 The child has lost 25–40% of the blood volume.
3 Meningococcal septicaemia: penicillin
Opiate poisoning: naloxone
Anaphylaxis: adrenaline
Wheezing: salbutamol
Carbon monoxide poisoning: high percentage oxygen
4 Dissociative shock should be treated with high percentage oxygen and rapid transfer to hospital. Carbon monoxide poisoning is a common cause.
5 Pulse oximetry may be unreliable in severe anaemia, shock, bright sunlight, hypothermia, and carbon monoxide poisoning.

CHAPTER 12: THE STRUCTURED APPROACH TO THE SERIOUSLY INJURED CHILD

1 The heart rate, pulse volume, capillary refill time, skin colour, respiratory rate, and mental status (with or without blood pressure) may be useful in estimating the degree of shock.
2 A jaw thrust, suction, oropharyngeal airway, endotracheal intubation, or surgical airway may be indicated to secure the airway. The most simple should be tried first.
3 Patients should be examined by:
Inspection
Palpation
Percussion and
Auscultation (Listening)

CHAPTER 13: TREATING SERIOUSLY INJURED CHILDREN

Section 13.1

1 Primary brain damage may be caused by cerebral lacerations, contusions, dural sac tears or diffuse axonal injury.

2 A potentially serious head injury may be suggested by the mechanism of injury suggesting substantial force, a history of loss of consciousness, children who have an altered level of response when examined, neurological symptoms, and signs or evidence of a penetrating head injury.

3 The most important indicator of spinal injury is the mechanism of injury.

4 Potential spinal trauma should be suspected when there is back or neck pain during movement or at rest, tenderness over the spine, on palpation, deformity or swelling, guarding of the neck or back or tingling, "pins and needles" or numbness.

Section 13.2

1 Life threatening injuries of the chest are:
Tension pneumothorax
Massive haemothorax
Open pneumothorax
Cardiac tamponade
Flail chest
Other major injuries include tracheobronchial rupture, ruptured diaphragm, and disruption of the great vessels.

2 All serious chest injuries require high concentration oxygen and urgent transfer to hospital.

3 The abdomen should be inspected for bruising, lacerations, and penetrating wounds, and palpated for tenderness and rigidity.

Section 13.3

1 The two types of life threatening extremity injury are traumatic amputation and massive open long bone fractures.

2 A child's bone has ongoing growth from the physis. In addition, the bone is structured such that it allows much more deformation without fracture and more absorption of force. Healing is rapid and remodelling can occur.

3 The primary concern, as always, is safety—of self, the scene, and then the patient.

4 Good prognostic factors in near drowned children are a time to first gasp of less than 3 minutes after the onset of BLS, and a core temperature of less than 33°C.

Index

Page numbers in **bold** type refer to figures; those in *italics* refer to tables or boxed text